This report evaluates the incidence of selected adverse birth outcomes in a Los Angeles population receiving some reclaimed water (i.e., wastewater that has been converted to reusable water through a multistep treatment process) in its residential water supply compared to a similar population that does not receive reclaimed water. The groundwater basin in the Montebello Forebay area of Los Angeles County has been replenished with some reclaimed water since 1962. RAND's epidemiologic assessment of the process of groundwater recharge with reclaimed water is part of an ongoing effort to monitor the health of those consuming reclaimed water in Los Angeles County. The report compares rates of low birth weight, very low birth weight, preterm birth, infant mortality, and birth defects in an area receiving reclaimed water and a matched control area not receiving reclaimed water in Los Angeles County. This report complements the results of a recent study of cancer incidence, mortality, and infectious disease in the Montebello Forebay population (Sloss et al., 1996). The results will be considered in the decisions made by regulatory agencies regarding the use of reclaimed water to augment drinking water supplies. This assessment was conducted by RAND for the Water Replenishment District of Southern California.

The report should be of interest to those concerned with issues related to water quality, including water industry personnel, and those in the field of public health.

Groundwater Recharge with Reclaimed Water

*Birth Outcomes
in Los Angeles County,
1982–1993*

Elizabeth M. Sloss

Daniel F. McCaffrey

Ronald D. Fricker

Sandra A. Geschwind

Beate R. Ritz

Prepared for the Water Replenishment District of Southern California

RAND

CONTENTS

FIGURES

This report describes an epidemiologic study designed to measure the association between adverse birth outcomes and residence in an area with some reclaimed water in the drinking water supply. This study focuses on a population living in the Montebello Forebay region of eastern Los Angeles County, California. In this area, reclaimed water has been used in conjunction with other water sources to recharge the groundwater basin since 1962. We analyzed data on adverse birth outcomes among infants born between 1982 and 1993 to women living in this area, a period from 20 to 30 years after groundwater recharge with reclaimed water was initiated in the Montebello Forebay. This report updates the results of earlier studies of birth outcomes occurring in the Montebello Forebay population between 1969 and 1980 (Frerichs et al., 1981, 1982b, 1983). These studies found no association between reclaimed water and higher rates of low birth weight, infant mortality, and congenital malformations recorded at the time of birth. The results in this report also complement a recent epidemiologic study (Sloss et al., 1996) that investigated patterns of cancer incidence, mortality, and infectious diseases from 1987 to 1991 in the Montebello Forebay region of Los Angeles County.

Using a cohort study design with a ZIP-code-level measure of exposure, this report examines the association between residence in an area with reclaimed water and several adverse birth outcomes. Existing data on births (1982–1993 birth certificates), infant deaths (1982–1993 birth and death certificates), and birth defects (1990–1993 registry data from the California Birth Defects Monitoring Program) were analyzed. Outcome categories included low birth weight, very low birth weight, preterm birth, infant mortality, and 19 categories of birth defects (all birth defects, excluding syndromes; all chromosomal syndromes; all syndromes other than chromosomal; and 16 specific types of birth defects). Rates of the adverse birth outcomes were compared between the area in eastern Los Angeles County with reclaimed water and a matched control area in Los Angeles County receiving no reclaimed water. Each birth was assigned to an exposure group based on the average annual percentage of reclaimed water in water supplied by systems serving the ZIP code. Logistic regression methods were used to generate odds ratios and confidence intervals to compare outcome rates in the reclaimed water and control groups.

The pattern of results indicates that rates of the prenatal development outcomes and infant mortality between 1982 and 1993, and rates of all types of birth defects between 1990 and 1993 were similar in the reclaimed water and control groups.

Some outcome rates were significantly higher and others were significantly lower for the reclaimed water groups compared to the control group. The results in this report, however, do not generally support the hypothesis of an association between residence in an area receiving reclaimed water and higher rates of these outcomes or a dose-response relationship between reclaimed water and the rate of these outcomes.

The limitations of epidemiologic methods make drawing conclusions about the effects of reclaimed water on adverse birth outcomes difficult. Personal characteristics that might affect the outcomes in this report—such as cigarette smoking, alcohol consumption, and occupational exposure—were assumed to be equal in the reclaimed water and control groups, but we could not control these in the analysis. If the distribution of these factors differs substantially between the reclaimed water and control groups, the pattern of results may be attributable to these differences or to other uncontrolled factors. In addition, exposure to reclaimed water may be misclassified because we used a surrogate measure of exposure—residence in an area receiving reclaimed water at the time of birth—rather than data on individual exposure throughout pregnancy. Individual exposure would be determined by many factors, including volume of tap water consumed, time spent away from home, and consumption of bottled water and other beverages. Finally, the high population mobility in Los Angeles County may make detecting an effect more difficult. Despite their limitations, the patterns of results in this report provide little evidence of an association between reclaimed water and adverse birth outcomes. The results of this or any other epidemiologic study cannot certify that reclaimed water has no effect on human health. We can conclude, however, that if reclaimed water is causing higher rates of any of these adverse birth outcomes, the increased risk is likely to be small.

We would like to acknowledge the efforts of many people inside and outside RAND without whom this research would not have been possible. We would like to thank Suzanne Polich for her outstanding work in preparing and managing the data files and Deborah Wesley for analyzing data from the 1990 Census. We would also like to thank our RAND colleague, Roy Gates, for his assistance in creating and extracting data from numerous Geographic Information System files required by this study. Harold Morgan, Richard Anderson, and others at Bookman-Edmonston Engineering, Inc., provided RAND with the data on the percentage of reclaimed water served to residents of the Montebello Forebay. Lisa Croen and John Harris of the California Birth Defects Monitoring Program arranged for RAND's use of the birth defects data.

We would also like to acknowledge the contributions of others. We thank David Savitz and Gayle Windham for excellent suggestions based on their reviews of an earlier draft. The report also incorporates the thoughtful comments of Rodger Baird and Margaret Nellor of the County Sanitation Districts of Los Angeles County and Lisa Croen of the California Birth Defects Monitoring Program. In addition, we appreciate the guidance throughout the study of the members of the advisory committee: Rodger Baird, Lisa Croen, Margaret Nellor, Harold Morgan, and Rick Sakaji and Gary Yamamoto of the California Department of Health Services. Finally, we are grateful to the Water Replenishment District of Southern California for support and assistance throughout this project, with special thanks to our project officers, Mario Garcia and Jim Leserman.

BPA	British Paediatric Association
CBDMP	California Birth Defects Monitoring Program
CI	Confidence interval
CNS	Central nervous system
COD	Chemical oxygen demand
DHS	(California) Department of Health Services
DWR	(California) Department of Water Resources
GAM	Generalized additive model
GEE	Generalized estimating equation
LBW	Low birth weight
MCL	Maximum contaminant level
MMWR	Mortality and Morbidity Weekly Review
MWD	Metropolitan Water District (Southern California)
NRC	National Research Council
NTD	Neural tube defect
ppb	Parts per billion
ppm	Parts per million
SMR	Standardized mortality ratio
SPMR	Standardized proportionate mortality ratio
THM	Trihalomethane
TTHM	Total THM
TOC	Total organic carbon
VOC	Volatile organic compound
WRP	Water reclamation plant

Chapter One

INTRODUCTION

This report describes an epidemiologic study designed to measure the association between adverse birth outcomes and residence in an area with some reclaimed water in its drinking water supply.[1] In the Montebello Forebay region of eastern Los Angeles County, California, reclaimed water has been used with other water sources to recharge the groundwater basin since 1962. This report is part of an ongoing effort to monitor all aspects of the health of the population in this area. Previous epidemiologic studies of birth outcomes occurring in the Montebello Forebay population between 1969 and 1980 found no association between reclaimed water and higher rates of low birth weight, infant mortality, and congenital malformations recorded at the time of birth (Frerichs et al., 1981, 1982a, 1982b, 1983; Frerichs, 1984; Nellor et al., 1984).

This report updates the results of these earlier studies by focusing on the years 1982 through 1993 (the most recently available data), a period during which both the percentage of reclaimed water and the number of areas with reclaimed water in the water supply have increased substantially. The results in this report complement another epidemiologic study that investigated patterns of cancer incidence, mortality, and infectious diseases from 1987 to 1991 in the Montebello Forebay region (Sloss et al., 1996).

In addition to these epidemiologic studies, a number of studies in other disciplines have been completed in the past 15 years on topics related to the health effects of using reclaimed water for potable purposes (National Research Council, 1998). Most of these studies have compared reclaimed and conventional drinking water sources. The studies have addressed a variety of topics, including developing and testing new methods for identifying organic chemicals and microbiological agents in reclaimed water and whole-animal toxicological studies. These studies have not detected any significant health effects from chemical compounds or infectious disease agents in reclaimed water. Together with the results from the epidemiologic studies, this leads to the conclusion that the quality of highly treated reclaimed water is as "safe" as other drinking water sources for the measures considered. Limitations in the meth-

---

[1]Water systems in the Montebello Forebay serve water that has been recharged with reclaimed water, resulting in an estimated percentage of reclaimed water between 1 and 38 percent (see Chapter Three, "Methods"). None of the water systems serve more reclaimed water than this; therefore, here we use the term "some reclaimed water." Throughout the rest of the report, we have shortened the term describing these water supplies to "reclaimed water."

ods used in all these investigations, however, have led many scientists to refrain from endorsing planned potable reuse as completely free of adverse health effects. The results in this report will be considered by regulatory agencies in making decisions regarding the safety of groundwater recharge with reclaimed water. Information from this and previous studies contributes to the continuing debate regarding the effects on human health of augmenting drinking water supplies with reclaimed water.

The rest of this chapter summarizes the treatment process of water reclamation, the regulatory process for use of reclaimed water in California, and previous research on health effects related to reclaimed water. Most of this background material has been presented previously (Sloss et al., 1996) but is repeated here to help the reader better understand the remainder of the report.

BACKGROUND

In recent decades, increasing populations in urban areas and a dwindling number of new water sources have led to increased conservation and reuse of water (National Research Council, 1998). Newer municipal areas have initiated reuse of wastewater for nonpotable purposes, such as irrigation of parks and golf courses. A smaller number of areas have started or are considering augmenting the potable water supply with highly treated wastewater. In many areas of the United States, the best available sources of water have been developed to the maximum possible extent, yet still fall short of the demand. This has motivated municipalities to consider augmenting their drinking water supplies in creative and inexpensive ways.

Southern California, with its large population and limited local water supplies, has had an ongoing need for alternative sources of water over the past several decades. The shortage of local water has been addressed in two ways: by importing water from other areas and by using water from aquifers, known as groundwater. About two-thirds of Southern California's water is imported from areas up to 500 miles away. The remaining one-third is pumped from the groundwater basins throughout the area (Nellor et al., 1984).

Both solutions to the water shortage might have negative consequences. Importing water, in addition to being expensive, raises concerns about the effect on the environment surrounding the source waters. On the other hand, natural groundwater supplies are limited in such semiarid areas as Southern California. Use of groundwater, therefore, can rapidly deplete the underground supplies or may require ongoing artificial replenishment. In many places in California, the use of groundwater has led to overdraft conditions and saltwater intrusion, with subsequent discontinuation of groundwater extraction. Some areas in Southern California have chosen to replenish the groundwater with water from other sources. The process of replacing water in aquifers is known as groundwater recharge (Nellor et al., 1984).

This report adds information to the debate regarding the possible effects on human health of using reclaimed water to recharge a groundwater basin. The use of reclaimed water for groundwater recharge began in the Montebello Forebay region in 1962. Over the past 30 years, the volume of reclaimed water used to replenish the Montebello Forebay basin has increased from 12,000 acre-feet per year in 1962 to 50,000 acre-feet per year in the mid-1980s to a maximum of 60,000 acre-feet per year in the early 1990s. Other water sources have also been used to recharge the basin, including local storm water runoff and imported surface water from the Colorado River and State Water Project (Nellor et al., 1984).

Wastewater Reuse

Throughout history, man has discharged waste matter into bodies of water. With small numbers of humans and large volumes of water, nature degraded the waste without degrading the quality of the water. As the waste volume increased, the delicate balance in these waters shifted, leading to pollution. Now, in many places in the United States, reclaiming water for reuse is a carefully monitored treatment process.[2]

Currently, wastewater is reused in several ways throughout the United States (Blanton, 1992). *Direct reuse* consists of treated wastewater delivered to the user directly by pipe or through a reservoir. In the United States, direct reuse is restricted to nonpotable uses, such as industrial processes, recreational facilities, and irrigation. Untreated household wastewater (other than toilet wastewater), called "gray water," is used for domestic irrigation and toilet flushing. All of these methods of reusing water are called *intentional direct reuse for nonpotable purposes*.

When treated and untreated wastewater is returned to a river or other body of water, it is often inadvertently withdrawn from these sources for use. This type of *indirect* reuse commonly occurs in rivers. If the body of water both receives wastewater and is the source of drinking water, this unplanned and uncontrolled reuse is called *unintentional indirect reuse. Intentional indirect reuse of reclaimed wastewater for potable purposes* is a term reserved for planned groundwater recharge with extensively treated tertiary effluents from water reclamation plants (Blanton, 1992).

Intentional indirect potable reuse takes place at numerous locations throughout the United States, of which Hamann et al. (1991) have described five. One of these, the Montebello Forebay (Whittier Narrows Water Reclamation Plant) in Los Angeles County, California, is the focus of this report. Two of the other sites are also in California: Water Factory 21 in Orange County and the Tahoe-Truckee Sanitation Agency Water Reclamation Plant in Nevada County. The remaining two sites are the Upper Occoquan Sewage Authority (UOSA) Water Reclamation Plant in Fairfax County, Virginia, and the Fred Hervey Water Reclamation Plant in El Paso County, Texas.

Residents of other areas of the United States may be exposed to much higher percentages of reclaimed water in their household supplies than those areas with inten-

---

[2]Reuse refers to a system in which water is used more than once by humans. Reclamation or reclaiming water refers to the process of treating the water to make it suitable for reuse by humans.

tional indirect reuse of reclaimed water (Robeck et al., 1987). Some river water may contain much higher percentages of "reclaimed water" than water from groundwater basins replenished with reclaimed water. For example, residents of Cincinnati and New Orleans use river water downstream from major drainage basins that collect from numerous municipal and industrial outflows. Although such water is not reclaimed using a formal treatment process and is not reused in an "intentional" manner, it is nonetheless reclaimed and reused water. Use of reclaimed water under these circumstances is not subject to the same close scrutiny as the intentional reuse of deliberately reclaimed water that is practiced in the Montebello Forebay. Studying such populations, however, might provide information on a related topic: the health effects of drinking unintentionally reclaimed and reused water.

Treatment of Reclaimed Water

The reclaimed water used for recharging the Montebello Forebay groundwater basin is derived from municipal wastewater that has been used in households, workplaces, and industries. This wastewater flows from its point of use through clay or concrete pipes to treatment plants. The process used to treat the wastewater at these plants essentially duplicates and accelerates what occurs in nature. A multistep treatment process is used to convert the wastewater to reusable water (Figure 1.1).

In a process similar to that of other sewage treatment plants, the water reclamation plants operated by the Los Angeles County Sanitation Districts (Sanitation Districts) start their wastewater treatment with primary and secondary treatment. The wastewater is transported from the sewer lines into a long concrete tank for its primary treatment. During primary treatment, sand, gravel, and other inorganic materials are allowed to settle out in tanks (sedimentation). Secondary treatment depends on biological processes to digest much of the remaining organic waste. Bacteria and other microorganisms break down the organic material in an aerated tank to produce harmless by-products such as carbon dioxide and water. After this process is completed, the bacteria-laden sludge is separated from the remaining liquid by settling. During primary and secondary treatment, suspended solids are reduced by about 90 percent. Secondary treatment is effective in reducing the number of viruses and bacteria and removing metals (through solids separation) and organic chemicals (through biodegradation). The next stage of treatment at the water reclamation plants goes beyond what sewage treatment plants normally provide. This stage, called tertiary treatment, consists of mono- or dual-media filtration. Disinfection is achieved through chlorination. Treatment with chlorine is essential for controlling infectious agents in the reclaimed wastewater.

Very few halogenated organic compounds occur in reclaimed water from the Sanitation Districts' plants. Concentrations for trihalomethanes (THMs) are typically less than 5 µg/l (Montebello Forebay Groundwater Recharge Engineering Report, 1997). Halogenated organics (e.g., THMs) are formed during a reaction between chlorine and organic material in the water and have been associated with health risks in some studies (Robeck et al., 1987). The potential to form such compounds depends large-

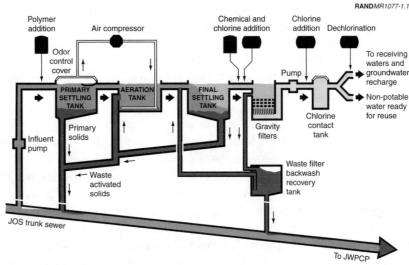

SOURCE: County Sanitation Districts of Los Angeles County.

Figure 1.1—Treatment Process in Los Angeles County Sanitation Districts' Water Reclamation Plants

ly on the absence of ammonia. Because the effluent from the Los Angeles County reclamation plants contains ammonia, few halogenated organics are formed. To prevent production of halogenated organics after leaving the treatment plant, the water is dechlorinated.

Assuming the wastewater treatment plants perform reliably, Robeck et al. (1987) claim that extensively treated wastewater might well be of better quality than many surface waters commonly used as sources of drinking water.

Reclaimed Water in the Montebello Forebay

The reclaimed water used for groundwater recharge in the Montebello Forebay is currently produced by three treatment plants. From 1962 until 1973, the Whittier Narrows Water Reclamation Plant (WRP) was the sole provider of reclaimed water in the form of disinfected secondary effluent. In 1973, the San Jose Creek Water Reclamation Plant began supplying secondary effluent for recharge. Some surplus effluent from a third treatment plant, the Pomona WRP, is released to the San Jose Wash, which ultimately flows to the San Gabriel River and becomes an incidental source for recharge in the Montebello Forebay. In 1978, all three WRPs added tertiary treatment with mono- or dual-media filtration and chlorination/dechlorination to their treatment regime.

After leaving the reclamation plants, the reclaimed water is conveyed to spreading areas whereby it can be delivered to one of several destinations. Effluent from the Whittier Narrows WRP can be delivered to the Rio Hondo spreading grounds from either of two discharge points. Alternatively, Whittier Narrows effluent is carried via pipeline from the plant to the San Gabriel River. San Jose Creek WRP effluent usually is conveyed through a pipeline to the San Gabriel River. From this point, water can either be released for spreading in the unlined San Gabriel River channel or in the adjacent spreading grounds. Effluent from the San Jose Creek WRP also can be released to the San Jose Wash and then be delivered either to the San Gabriel River or conveyed across the Whittier Narrows to the Rio Hondo, where it can be diverted into the Rio Hondo spreading grounds.

The reclaimed water blends with other sources of water in the aquifers. The regulatory agency responsible for overseeing the spreading operations (the Regional Water Quality Control Board) requires that reclaimed water must blend with other sources but that this may occur as the reclaimed water moves underground throughout the aquifers. No regulatory provisions require blending to take place at the surface prior to groundwater recharge. Only a portion of recharged waters can consist of reclaimed water, with limitations based on both annual and three-year running averages. No more than 50 percent of recharged water in any one year can consist of reclaimed water. On a running three-year-average basis, no more than 35 percent of total recharge to the Montebello Forebay can consist of reclaimed water. In actual volume, reclaimed water can amount to no more than 60,000 acre-feet annually and no more than 150,000 acre-feet over a running three-year period. Mixing the sources used for groundwater recharge is important in reducing the concentration of any unidentified contaminants that might be present in any one of the sources (Nellor et al., 1984).

In the process of groundwater recharge, the water percolates through an unsaturated zone of soil ranging in average thickness of about 10 to 40 feet before reaching the groundwater table. The process of "surface spreading"[3] takes place in several areas, including two areas of spreading ground facilities (San Gabriel River and Rio Hondo) and in the unlined San Gabriel River channel. These areas together cover some 700 wetted acres of land in the Montebello Forebay recharge operation. The usual spreading schedule consists of a repeated 21-day cycle of flooding and drying. The cycle consists of five days of flooding during which water is piped into the basins and maintained at a constant depth. The flow is then discontinued, followed by 16 days during which the basins are allowed to drain and dry out. This cycle of wet and dry maintains the proper conditions for the percolation process (Crook et al, 1990; Nellor et al., 1984). During percolation, trace organic compounds are reduced substantially, primarily through biodegradation, aided somewhat by adsorption and volatilization (Nellor et al., 1984).

Regulation of Reclaimed Water Use in California

In the early 1970s, the State Water Resources Control Board (SWRCB) oversaw the development of long-range plans for water basins throughout California. These plans identified more than 30 projects entailing groundwater recharge, some of

---

[3] *Surface spreading* is a method of groundwater recharge in which the water travels from the land surface to the aquifer by infiltration and percolation through the soil. *Spreading basins* are the areas of land designated for surface spreading (Crook et al., 1992).

which proposed augmenting domestic water sources with reclaimed water (Crook et al., 1990). In response to these plans, the California Department of Health Services (DHS) issued a position statement in 1973 regarding the proposed uses of reclaimed water.

In this position statement, the DHS outlined guidelines for use of reclaimed water, including what it considered inappropriate uses, such as direct addition of reclaimed water into domestic water supplies, and direct injection into groundwater (i.e., without percolation). As justification for these recommendations, the document cites the possibility of long-term health effects associated with organic material remaining in reclaimed water after treatment. With regard to surface spreading of reclaimed water, it stated that the use of surface spreading seems promising; the health effects of surface spreading are unknown; if recharge with reclaimed water is associated with adverse effects, groundwater basins might have to be closed; setting an "acceptable" level of reclaimed water was not possible without more information; and recharge of large basins with a relatively small volume of reclaimed water might be acceptable (Crook et al., 1990). In conclusion, the report stated that surface spreading of reclaimed water might be an option.

In 1975, three of California's state agencies—DHS, SWRCB, and the Department of Water Resources (DWR)—formed a Consulting Panel on the Health Aspects of Wastewater Reclamation for Groundwater Recharge following the issuance of the DHS position statement (Crook et al., 1990). The panel was supposed to recommend research related to reclaimed water aimed at two objectives. First, the research should enable the DHS to formulate reasonable criteria for groundwater recharge with reclaimed water. Second, the recommended research should help the DWR and SWRCB to design and initiate programs that would encourage the use of reclaimed water in line with these criteria.

The Consulting Panel focused on research tasks related to groundwater recharge with reclaimed water by surface spreading. The panel recommended that studies be conducted to elucidate health effects and estimate any health risk (Crook et al., 1990). The studies should be aimed at characterizing any contaminants, exploring the toxicology, and studying the epidemiology of the exposed populations. The panel suggested that data for these studies should be derived from ongoing projects that were using reclaimed water, as well as new projects that could be conducted under more controlled conditions.

In 1976, the DHS wrote draft regulations for groundwater recharge with reclaimed water by surface spreading (Crook et al., 1990). The objective of the proposed regulations was to eliminate stable organic chemicals from the water. The draft regulations specified that wastewater should undergo secondary treatment followed by carbon adsorption and percolation through 10 feet of soil. Water quality standards were proposed for reclaimed water for a number of constituents: inorganic chemicals, pesticides, radioactivity, chemical oxygen demand (COD), and total organic carbon (TOC). Separate standards were proposed for the quality of the groundwater receiving the reclaimed water. The draft regulations specified that reclaimed water could not exceed 50 percent of all water spread in a 12-month period and that it should remain underground for one year before being pumped out. The proposed regulations also requested an effluent monitoring program, hydrogeology and spreading reports, an industrial monitoring program, contingency plans, and an on-going program to monitor the health of populations receiving reclaimed water. The breadth of these draft regulations made the implementation of the complete set too costly and unmanageable. They were not adopted as statewide criteria but rather were recommended as guidelines for new groundwater recharge projects (Crook et al., 1990).

These wastewater reclamation criteria were revised by the DHS in 1978 (Crook et al., 1990). The revision targeted the quality of reclaimed water to be used to recharge aquifers for domestic water supplies, requiring that the quality "fully protect public health." DHS also suggested that each recharge project be considered based on its individual characteristics, including treatment, quality and volume of effluent, spreading grounds, soil for percolation, hydrogeology, time in aquifer, and time to withdrawal. The criteria were also amended to require a DHS-held public hearing prior to approval of a new project.

The pressure to use reclaimed water in Southern California heightened following the 1976–1977 drought. The recommendations of the Consulting Panel, however, deterred water officials from starting new projects or expanding existing projects. In 1978, a study of health effects related to groundwater recharge with reclaimed water (called the Health Effects Study) was initiated by the Sanitation District. This study was completed over a five-year period at a cost of $1.4 million (Crook et al., 1990). The design and results of this study are reported in detail in the final report (Nellor et al., 1984) and summarized in the next section.

Health Effects Study

The goal of the Health Effects Study was to compile information for health and regulatory authorities who would be making decisions about the use of reclaimed water in California. One of these decisions was whether reclaimed water for groundwater recharge in the Montebello Forebay should be maintained at the same level, increased, or decreased. The information collected during the study had two objectives: to assess whether groundwater recharge with reclaimed water had affected the groundwater quality or human health adversely and to compare the effects of various water sources used for recharge on groundwater quality (Nellor et al., 1984).

The study's research tasks included (1) water-quality characterizations of groundwater in the Montebello Forebay basin, reclaimed water the Sanitation District treatment plants, and other recharge sources; (2) toxicological and chemical studies of the same water sources; (3) studies to determine the effect of percolation on the quality of reclaimed water; (4) hydrogeological studies to establish movement of reclaimed water within the groundwater basin; and (5) epidemiologic studies of populations living in areas served reclaimed water. The major findings of the study are summarized below, drawing heavily from the final report by Nellor et al. (1984). Following this subsection is a summary of the findings and recommendations of a Scientific Advisory Panel appointed by the State of California to review the status of information on health, technology, and monitoring aspects of recharging ground-water with reclaimed water.

Water Quality Characterization. The water quality characterization is based on 56 samples from the following sites in the Montebello Forebay:

- 24 unchlorinated samples from eight wells (groundwater)
- Six chlorinated samples from two wells (groundwater)
- Three unchlorinated secondary effluent samples from a water reclamation plant (reclaimed water)
- Three chlorinated secondary effluent samples from a water reclamation plant (reclaimed water)
- Eight chlorinated/dechlorinated tertiary effluent samples from a water recla-mation plant (reclaimed water)
- Three samples from imported Colorado River water (imported water)
- Three samples from imported State Project water (imported water)
- Six storm water samples (storm water).

Groundwater and reclaimed water met all federal drinking water regulations for microorganisms and for organic and inorganic chemicals. The concentration of unregulated "health-significant" organic compounds in some samples of reclaimed water and storm water exceeded guidelines set by DHS. The levels of such com-pounds in groundwater and imported water, however, did not exceed these limits.

The water quality characterization studies revealed that a group of nontargeted industrial organics and metabolic by-products (e.g., phthalates, solvents, and petroleum by-products) were found at a significantly higher concentration in both reclaimed water and storm water. Overall, in the 1984 Health Effects Study, only about 10 percent of the organic matter contained in reclaimed water was identified.

The organic complexity of the groundwater appeared to be related to the proximity of the sampling site to industrial areas. Its THM concentration was influenced by chlorination practices at the wells. The average groundwater concentration of sol-vents and pesticides was below estimated carcinogenic risk levels. Industrial organ-ics were present in all groundwater samples, leading to the conclusion that water supplies need to be protected from improper handling of chemicals—mainly improper industrial waste disposal.

Virus Sampling. No viruses were recovered from groundwater (110 samples) or the chlorinated tertiary effluents of the four California wastewater treatment facilities (174 samples) analyzed for the study.

Toxicology and Trace Organics Studies. Ninety samples were collected and pre-pared for the toxicology and trace organics studies. All percolation sources—reclaimed water, storm water, and imported water—as well as unchlorinated and chlorinated well water were analyzed for the compounds listed in Table 1.1 (Nellor et al., 1984). The levels of some trace organic compounds in reclaimed water, imported water, and storm water exceeded the "theoretical lifetime risk assessment" values from the (at the time) proposed Environmental Protection Agency (EPA) water quality criteria. The average concentrations of organic compounds in *groundwater*, however, did not exceed these values. The organic compounds detected in well water originated in all three percolation sources and from the chlorination practices at the wells. The following compounds were detected in the specified sources:

Surface runoff water: tetrachloroethylene, atrazine, simazine, propazine, chlorinated phenols, phenylacetic acid, and phthalates.

Reclaimed water: methylene chloride, chloroform, trichloroethylene, tetrachloroethylene, chlorinated phenols, and phthalates.

Water imported from the Colorado River: THMs and phthalates.

Chlorination practices: THMs.

Although these compounds were above the detection limits, their levels were insignificant relative to the EPA's maximum contaminant levels, the National Academy of Sciences' "suggested no adverse response levels," and the California State Department of Health Services' "action levels" (Nellor et al., 1984).

In the toxicology studies, water concentrates from the four water treatment plants were tested with a fortified Ames Salmonella Microsome Mutagen Assay. The mutagenicity of the reclaimed water was found to be intermediate between the high mutagenicity of storm runoff and dry weather runoff and the low mutagenicity of imported Colorado River water (Robeck et al., 1987). Mammalian cell assays were performed to detect carcinogenic action. None was detected for these samples.

Table 1.1

Compounds in Target Organic Analyses in the Health Effects Study

Target Compounds	
Vinyl chloride	DDT
Methylene chloride	Dieldrin
Chloroform	Aldrin
Bromodichloromethane	Lindane
Dibromochloromethane	Atrazine
Bromoform	Simazine
Carbon tetrachloride	Pentachlorophenol
1,1-dichloroethane	Trichlorobiphenyls (as total PCB)
1,2-dichloroethane	Tetrachlorobiphenyls (as total PCB)
1,1,2-trichloroethane	Trichlorobenzene (1,2,4-isomer)
Trichloroethylene	Trichlorophenol (2,4,6-isomer)
Tetrachloroethylene	Trichlorophenol (2,4,5-isomer)
Chlorobenzene	Bis (2-ethylhexyl) phthalate
1,4-dichlorobenzene	Phenylacetic acid
1,2-dichlorobenzene	Fluoranthene
Benzene	Phenanthrene
Toluene	Benzo(a)pyrene

According to chemical and biological assays, the compounds responsible for the mutagenicity may have been organic halides and epoxides. Although some compounds in these classes are known mutagens and animal carcinogens, the significance of the mutagenicity finding was limited by the lack of precise identification of the compounds. The occurrence and action of such compounds may not be limited to the Montebello Forebay recharge project. Compounds similar to these may be responsible for the low-level mutagenicity found in drinking water samples nationwide.

The possibility of interactions, and the fact that many organic substances in reclaimed water are unknown or not yet identifiable, stimulated a shift from trying to classify each single compound toxicologically to assessing the mutagenic and carcinogenic potential of concentrated samples of reclaimed water as a whole. The drawback of this procedure is that it limits the assessment of the quality of reclaimed water to that produced by a specific treatment plant at only one point in time; in fact the quality of reclaimed water might vary with treatment practices as well as with the quality of the influent water. Although the results of the Ames test have not demonstrated correlations with possible health effects in humans, this test is a useful screening tool for detecting the presence of organics capable of causing damage to genetic material (as possible carcinogens) in complex organic mixtures (Nellor et al., 1984).

Percolation Study. A separate percolation study was conducted to determine possible changes in water quality resulting from the percolation of water through soil. It concluded that soil percolation did not consistently remove target trace organics from reclaimed water. Organic chemicals are biotransformed by microorganisms residing in subsurface material. The rate and extent of such transformation, however, are dependent on the availability of organisms and their metabolic requirements with respect to oxygen, pH, and mineral nutrients. The adsorption capacity of soil is variable; materials introduced by repeated spreading of treated wastewater change the geochemical properties of the subsurface environment over time.

Epidemiology Studies. The epidemiologic studies conducted as part of the Health Effects Study investigated both short- and long-term health effects of reclaimed water, including occurrence of infectious diseases, adverse birth outcomes, and cancer incidence (Frerichs et al., 1981, 1982b, 1983). The epidemiologic studies used two general approaches: geographic comparison (or ecologic studies) and a household survey.

In the geographic comparison studies, routinely collected data were used to calculate average rates of mortality, cancer incidence, infectious disease, and adverse birth outcomes. Census tracts were classified into two exposure categories: high (greater than or equal to 5 percent reclaimed water during one or more years before 1970) or low (less than 5 percent reclaimed water for the years before 1970). Rates for the high and low reclaimed water areas were compared to rates in two control areas that had received no reclaimed water. This type of comparison was made for a broad range of health outcomes for three time periods: 1969–1971, 1972–1978, and 1979–1980.

The health outcomes included mortality (death from all causes, heart disease, stroke, all cancers, and cancers of the colon, stomach, bladder, and rectum), cancer incidence (all cancers and cancers of the colon, stomach, bladder, and rectum), infant and neonatal mortality, low birth weight and congenital malformations, and selected infectious diseases (including hepatitis A and shigella). The data were derived from the following sources:

- Mortality data: death certificates

- Cancer incidence data: cancer registry for Los Angeles County (University of Southern California Cancer Surveillance Program)

- Data on infant and neonatal mortality, low birth weight, and congenital malformations: birth and death certificates

- Infectious disease data: reportable disease information from the Los Angeles County Department of Health Services.

With few exceptions, only minor differences were found between the reclaimed water and control areas. The most noteworthy findings relate to higher standardized mortality ratios (SMRs) (or standardized proportionate mortality ratios, SPMRs) for rectal cancer in the reclaimed water census tracts. In the 1969–1971 period, the SMR was 1.67 (based on 18 deaths) in the "high" reclaimed water area and 1.17 (based on 45 deaths) in the "low" area. For the 1972–1978 period, the pattern was similar with an SPMR of 1.27 in the "high" area and 0.95 in the "low" area. In the 1979–1980 period, the SMR for rectal cancer *based on mortality data* was 1.52 (10 cases) for the "high" area and 0.63 in the "low" area (13 cases). For this same period, the SMR for rectal cancer *based on incidence data* from a Los Angeles County cancer registry was 0.82 for the high area and 0.60 for the low area, indicating no association between reclaimed water and rectal cancer incidence for the years studied. The authors stated that because cancer incidence data are considered a more sensitive indicator of the underlying occurrence of the disease than mortality data, the higher death rate due to rectal cancer "provides no reason for concern that exposure to reclaimed water is having a detrimental effect on the level of rectal cancer in the population." The authors also suggested that the difference between the mortality and incidence rates might be attributed to differences in coding practices between the local health care providers and the staff of the cancer registry (Frerichs et al., 1983).

A household survey was conducted in 1981 as part of the Health Effects epidemiologic study. The objective of the survey was to collect information on reproductive outcomes, consumption of water, and other personal characteristics from a sample of women 18 years of age and older. A total of 2,523 women were interviewed by telephone, 1,243 in the "high" reclaimed water area and 1,280 in the control area. Women in the reclaimed water and control areas reported 733 and 768 pregnancies, respectively. The analysis investigated possible differences between the women living in the two areas in spontaneous abortions and other adverse reproductive outcomes, bed-days, disability-days, perception of well-being, and health, controlling for personal health status and consumption of tap water. The study concluded that consumption of reclaimed water was not associated with a measurable increase in the rates of these outcomes.

Scientific Review of Health Effects Study

In 1986, the State of California appointed a Scientific Advisory Panel to review the status of information on health, technology, and monitoring aspects of recharging groundwater with reclaimed water (Robeck et al., 1987). As part of the review, the panel evaluated the design and methods used in the Health Effects Study. In its evaluation, the panel characterized the study as "thorough and well-conducted with state-of-the-art methodology." Concerns were expressed, however, regarding the limitations of the methods used in the Health Effects Study. The panel stated that the study showed that groundwater in the sampling sites is "contaminated with a variety of organic compounds of industrial, and perhaps treatment, origin," of which only about 10 percent were positively identified. Robeck et al. (1987) concluded that the data available from the characterization studies did not permit an unambiguous judgment regarding the likelihood that the majority of compounds present and of greatest health concern were identified. The panel also called for further work investigating the feasibility of a two-year oncogenicity protocol in rodents, using water samples or water concentrates. The panel's final concern related to the epidemiologic studies' ability to detect an effect on human cancer. Panel members felt that the high mobility of the population in Los Angeles County and long latent period for human cancers (20 or 30 years or longer) could render the epidemiologic results related to cancer inconclusive.

Among the panel's recommendations were the following: in any area, the highest-quality water available should be used for drinking; the Montebello Forebay Groundwater Replenishment Project should continue; surface spreading is preferable to injection as a means to recharge; reclaimed water should be disinfected, but disinfection should not produce harmful by-products; any new groundwater recharge project should conduct health surveillance of its population; concentrates of reclaimed water should be tested for small amounts of harmful substances; risk evaluation should be studied using animals in toxicology studies; and monitoring for chemicals should be continued (Robeck et al., 1987).

Rationale Behind Epidemiologic Studies of Reclaimed Water

Although the quality of reclaimed water is carefully monitored through extensive testing before and after recharge, epidemiologic studies add new and important information regarding the health effects of reclaimed water. First, studying the health of the population receiving reclaimed water allows evaluation of the effects of water quality even when detailed historical information on the levels of specific constituents is not available. Studies of water quality characterize samples of water at a single point in time or over a short period. These types of analyses cannot identify potentially harmful chemicals that may have been found in these water supplies months, years, or decades ago or contaminants that may occur sporadically. Second, epidemiologic investigations are one of the few ways to study the effects on human health directly. Although epidemiologic studies provide imperfect information, scientific studies in fields other than epidemiology often focus on information only indirectly related to human health. Water quality studies aim to identify individual chemicals, and toxicology studies attempt to estimate the biological effect of each chemical. Neither water quality studies nor toxicology studies, however, can predict the synergistic interaction of these chemicals within the human system or their cumulative effect over years of chronic low-level exposure. Other types of scientific studies can add valuable information to an epidemiologic assessment but cannot replace them (Ames, 1983).

Results of Study of Cancer, Mortality, and Infectious Disease

A previous study of the Montebello Forebay population was designed to measure the association between reclaimed water and cancer incidence, mortality, and incidence of infectious disease (Sloss et al., 1996). Existing data on cancer incidence (1987–1991 cancer registry records), mortality (1989–1991 death certificates), and infectious disease (1989–1990 reports to the Los Angeles County Health Department) were analyzed in conjunction with population counts from the 1990 Census. Rates of the health outcomes were compared in the reclaimed water and matched control areas. The analysis was based on routinely collected data on cancer incidence (all cancers and cancer of the bladder, colon, esophagus, kidney, liver, pancreas, rectum, and stomach), mortality (deaths due to all causes, heart disease, stroke, all cancer, and the same eight specific cancer sites), and infectious diseases (giardia, hepatitis A, salmonella, shigella, and several less common diseases). The census tracts being served reclaimed water were assigned to one of five exposure categories based on the percentage of reclaimed water in the drinking water supply. The maximum percentage of reclaimed water over the 30-year period (1960–1991) ranged between 0 and 31 percent for the 66 water systems in the Montebello Forebay. For most systems, the estimated annual percentage of reclaimed water increased consistently over the 30-year period. Multivariate Poisson regression methods were used to generate rate ratios and 95 percent confidence intervals.

The study concluded that between 1987 and 1991, almost 30 years after groundwater recharge with reclaimed water began, the rates of cancer, mortality, and infectious disease were similar in the area of Los Angeles County receiving reclaimed water and a control area not receiving reclaimed water. Rates of these health outcomes were also similar in areas receiving higher and lower percentages of reclaimed water. Regions with less reclaimed water tended to have higher rates of adverse health outcomes than regions with more reclaimed water. A few instances arose in which rates of disease or death were significantly higher in areas receiving reclaimed water than in the control area, including a significantly higher incidence rate of liver cancer in the area with the highest percentage of reclaimed water. The weakness of these associations, the absence of patterns consistent with a dose-response relationship, and the lack of scientific evidence to support a causal relationship between reclaimed water and liver cancer led to the conclusion that these results are most likely explained either by factors unrelated to reclaimed water or by chance occurrence. In conclusion, the results of the epidemiologic study by Sloss et al. (1996) did not provide evidence that supports an association between reclaimed water and higher rates of cancer, mortality, and infectious disease.

OVERVIEW OF REPORT

The objective of the study reported here was to measure the association between adverse birth outcomes and reclaimed water. This association is estimated based on an analysis of data on births occurring between 1982 and 1993 in two areas—both in Los Angeles County—one being served reclaimed water and the other, a matched control area served no reclaimed water.

This report provides a literature review, a detailed description of the methods employed, and the results of the study. Chapter Two reviews the scientific literature on adverse birth outcomes, focusing primarily on epidemiologic studies designed to measure the association between drinking water and low birth weight, birth defects, and spontaneous abortions. Chapter Three describes the study methods—the estimation of the population's exposure to reclaimed water, the selection of control locations, the sources of data on health outcomes and population characteristics, and the statistical techniques employed in the data analysis. Chapter Four presents the results of the study. It describes the location, size, and characteristics of the populations in the area receiving reclaimed water and in the control area, as well as the number and characteristics of the births that occurred in these areas throughout the study period. It also compares rates of adverse birth outcomes in the reclaimed water and control groups, reporting measures of association for the outcomes and reclaimed water. Chapter Five discusses the methods and results as well as the strengths and limitations of the study design.

Chapter Two

LITERATURE REVIEW

This chapter provides information from the scientific literature related to the adverse birth outcomes investigated: low birth weight, birth defects, and infant mortality. In the first section, we describe possible mechanisms for the effect of environmental exposures on the reproductive process. The following sections summarize available information on maternal and infant characteristics and other risk factors associated with adverse birth outcomes. In addition, we discuss published studies that measured the association between adverse birth outcomes and quality of drinking water based on specific constituents and source.

POSSIBLE MECHANISMS FOR ENVIRONMENTAL INFLUENCE ON ADVERSE BIRTH OUTCOMES

To hypothesize that adverse birth outcomes may stem from exposures to environmental chemicals, it is necessary to establish possible mechanisms for this type of effect. Such an effect might vary according to the timing of the exposure and thus the biologic target of the effect. Adverse effects of an environmental exposure are theoretically possible during two time frames within the reproductive cycle: prior to conception and during pregnancy.

Adverse effects before conception may occur in either the male or the nonpregnant female. In the male, exposures might cause genetic damage to the sperm, resulting in abnormal development of the fetus (Olshan and Faustmann, 1993). If stem cells are permanently harmed, they might produce genetically defective sperm indefinitely, that in turn might increase risk of abnormalities in the offspring (Scialli, 1992). In the female, an environmental exposure might cause genetic damage to the ovum before conception, and that in turn might result in a chromosomal defect in the offspring (Kline et al., 1989). These effects might not be observed until many years after the exposure.

Research related to the reproductive consequences of environmental exposures during pregnancy focuses on either the viability of the fetus or abnormalities observed in the infant after birth (Institute of Medicine, 1996). Depending on the timing of the harmful exposure and the effect of the exposure, a range of adverse outcomes might be observed. Exposure during pregnancy might result in fetal death, commonly called a miscarriage (early in pregnancy) or stillbirth (later). Nonfatal damage to the fetus during pregnancy might result in birth defects or low birth weight from impaired growth and development. Preterm delivery might result from either maternal health problems or developmental problems in the fetus.

Exposure to a single contaminant might induce a range of effects in different infants depending on a number of factors. A substance capable of acting at different stages of gestation might result in a different pathogenesis at each stage and, thus, produce different effects depending on the timing of exposure in relation to gestational age (Kline et al., 1989). Furthermore, if a common pathogenesis occurs at a fundamental molecular, cellular, or tissue level, it could produce seemingly diverse effects at higher levels of organization. This issue is difficult to study because information on the exact day or week of gestation when a pregnant woman was in contact with a specific chemical is rarely available. More often, exposure information is limited to trimester specification (i.e., first, second, or third).

IMPACT OF FETAL LOSS ON ADVERSE OUTCOMES AMONG LIVE BIRTHS

Infants born alive are the survivors of cohorts of conceptions that have experienced severe attrition. It has been estimated that between 17 and 50 percent of pregnancies end in spontaneous abortion before the seventeenth week of gestation (Kline et al., 1989, Weinberg et al., 1992). Weinberg et al. (1992) reported that about 68 percent of all pregnancy losses occur—mostly unrecognized by the woman—during the first 6 weeks after the last menstrual period. Another 25 percent of losses occur during early fetal life and are clinically recognizable. Abnormal embryonic and fetal development often result in spontaneous pregnancy terminations (Shiota, 1989).

The vulnerable period for the initiation of morphologic birth defects coincides with a period in early pregnancy during which pregnancy loss occurs most frequently (Kline et al., 1989). Severe, nonviable aberrations are a likely cause for such early loss. Thus, spontaneous abortions have a much higher rate of birth defects than those diagnosed at a later time in fetal development or after birth. In more than half of spontaneously aborted fetuses, a chromosome abnormality is present (Kline et al., 1989). In fact, only a small proportion of developmentally abnormal pregnancies result in live births. A larger proportion end in stillbirths, and most end in miscarriages (Kline et al., 1989). It has been estimated that more than 90 percent of chromosomal aberrations are lethal in utero (Kline et al., 1989). If an environmental agent causes a defect that renders a fetus nonviable, such an effect would not be detected by examining malformation rates at birth because the fetus will be miscarried early in pregnancy. Another selection mechanism that needs to be considered when studying adverse birth outcomes in a population of live births is the increasing rate of elective terminations that might result from increased screening for, and prenatal diagnosis of, neural tube defects in recent years (Forrester et al., 1998).

LOW BIRTH WEIGHT AND PRETERM BIRTH

Definitions related to low birth weight and preterm birth have evolved over the last few decades. Historically, infants with a birth weight less than or equal to 2,500 grams (about 5.5 pounds) were labeled "premature" (Berkowitz and Papiernik, 1993). Research showed, however, that within this group of small infants were three distinct subgroups: those born too early, those whose growth was retarded, and those born too early whose growth was retarded (Berkowitz and Papiernik, 1993). Based on this reasoning, two terms are now generally employed in the study of small infants: low birth weight and preterm birth. Low birth weight is defined as an infant weighing less than 2,500 grams at the time of birth, and preterm refers to an infant born at or before 37 weeks of gestation (World Health Organization, 1977). Using these definitions, 5.9 percent of the live births occurring in California in 1992 would be classified as low birth weight and 9.7 percent as preterm births (Riedmiller and Ficenec, 1994).

Intrauterine growth rates are measured by relating size of the infant at birth to its estimated gestational age. Thus, weight at birth is taken to imply a rate of growth during the gestational period beginning at conception. The most rapid weight gain occurs after the twentieth week of gestation, and exposures during the last trimester seem to be most relevant for asymmetric low birth weight (i.e., reduced weight, but not reduced length or head circumference). Preterm birth (i.e., birth occurring prior to the full gestational period) is another important cause for low weight at birth. Whether due to growth retardation or preterm birth, low birth weight increases the risk for perinatal mortality, and, thus, some authors prefer to make no distinction between these two etiologies of low birth weight.

Many factors are associated with low birth weight, including reduced length of gestation, female gender of the child, single motherhood, multiple births, maternal age (less than 15 years), nulliparity, short maternal height, and living at high altitudes (above 2,500 meters) (Kline et al., 1989; Defo and Partin, 1993; Pickering, 1987). Birth weight also varies with maternal race and ethnicity, with Hispanic and foreign-born women experiencing lower risk of low birth weight infants (Cobas et al., 1996; Singh and Yu, 1996; Hyman and Dussault, 1996; Cramer, 1995) and black and Asian-American women having a higher risk (Mor et al., 1995; Orr et al., 1996; Singh and Yu, 1994). Other risk factors for low birth weight include pregnancy complications (Lekea-Karanika and Tzoumaka-Bakoula, 1994; Schieve et al., 1994; Sharma et al., 1994), inadequate prenatal care (Barros et al., 1996), maternal cigarette smoking, exposure to second-hand smoke, and cocaine use (Lieberman et al., 1994; Kistin et al., 1996; Eskenazi et al., 1995; Zhang and Ratcliffe, 1993; Kurz et al., 1994), as are occupational noise and stress (Hartikainen et al., 1994; Nurminen, 1995; Xu et al., 1994; Ceron-Mireles et al., 1997). Some studies of air and soil contamination and low birth weight have found no association (Bhopal et al., 1994; Landgren, 1996; Sosniak et al., 1994; McMichael et al., 1986), and others have observed higher rates of low birth weight in residential areas with high levels of pollution (Sram et al., 1996; Berry and Bove, 1997).

BIRTH DEFECTS

The etiology of birth defects remains poorly understood with many questions remaining regarding the role of genetic and environmental factors. About 3 percent of all live births have one or more major birth defects (Hexter et al., 1990). Of these, about 10 percent can be attributed to a known teratogen (Hexter et al., 1990). Numerous factors have been identified as human teratogens (Table 2.1). These include maternal exposures to radiation, infections, maternal metabolic imbalance, drugs, and environmental chemicals. In addition, animal studies and/or human studies have identified a broad range of factors possibly associated with the occurrence of birth defects (Table 2.2).

Birth defect rates have been associated with socioeconomic status, ethnicity, maternal age, altitude, previous defects diagnosed in siblings, and parental consanguinity (Kline et al., 1989; Lopez-Camelo and Orioli, 1996; Pradat, 1994; Stoltenberg et al., 1997; Werler et al., 1992). Many of these factors, however, may be proxies for unidentified environmental, behavioral, or genetic factors. Environmental exposures, such as hazardous waste sites (Croen et al., 1997; Geschwind et al., 1992) and industrial facilities (Marshall et al., 1997), have also been associated with selected birth defects.

A protective effect for the occurrence of neural tube defects has been described for the first trimester use of vitamin E supplements (Sullivan, 1993) and folate (Werler et al., 1993) and has also been suggested for the use of multivitamins and congenital urinary tract defects (Li et al., 1995).

Table 2.1

Teratogenic Agents in Human Beings

Radiation	Drugs and Environmental Chemicals
Atomic weapons	(continued)
Radioiodine	Cyclophosphamide
Therapeutic	Diethylstilbestrol
Infections	Diphenylhydantoin
Cytomegalovirus (CMV)	Enalapril (renal failure)
Herpes virus hominis I and II	Etretinate
Parvovirus B-19 (Erthema infectiosum)	Iodides and goiter
Rubella virus	Lithium
Syphilis	Mercury, organic
Toxoplasmosis	Methimazole and scalp defects
Venezuelan equine encephalitis virus	Penicillamine
Maternal Metabolic Imbalance	13-cis-Retinoic acid (Isotretinoin and
Alcoholism	Accutane)
Cretinism, endemic	Tetracyclines
Diabetes	Thalidomide
Folic acid deficiency	Trimethadione
Hyperthermia	Valproic acid
Phenylketonuria	
Rheumatic disease and congenital heart block	
Virilizing tumors	
Drugs and Environmental Chemicals	
Aminopterin and methylaminopterin	
Busulfan	
Captopril (renal failure)	
Cholorophenyls	
Cocaine	
Coumarin anticoagulants	

SOURCE: Shepard, 1992.

Table 2.2

Possible and Unlikely Teratogens

Possible Teratogens	Unlikely Teratogens
Binge drinking	Agent Orange
Carbamazepine	Anesthetics
Chorionic villus sampling, early	Aspartame
Cigarette smoking	Aspirin
Disulfiram	Benedectin (antinauseants)
Ergotamine	Birth control pills
High vitamin A	Illicit drugs (marijuana, LSD)
Lead	Metronidazole (Flagyl)
Primidone	Oral contraceptives
Streptomycin	Rubella vaccine
Toluene abuse	Spermicides
Varicella virus	Video display screens
Zinc deficiency	

SOURCE: Shepard, 1992.

INFANT MORTALITY

Infant mortality, defined as deaths under one year of age, is a measure monitored closely as a public health indicator. Based on California births in 1992, the infant mortality rate was less than 1 percent (6.9 per 1,000 live births) (Riedmiller and Ficenec, 1994). Most of these deaths (61.0 percent) occurred among infants less than 28 days old. Of these, the five leading causes were perinatal conditions (including conditions related to low birth weight and preterm birth), congenital anomalies, sudden infant death syndrome, pneumonia and influenza, and accidents. Birth weight and number of defects are the strongest predictors of infant mortality (Druschel et al., 1996).

STUDIES OF DRINKING WATER AND ADVERSE BIRTH OUTCOMES

Overview of Study Designs and Methods

The influence of drinking water constituents on adverse pregnancy and birth outcomes has been studied in British, Australian, Canadian, and U.S. populations over several decades. Some investigations were initiated in response to public concern over local water contamination from an industrial source. Other studies are conducted to fulfill a more routine monitoring function in which investigators draw on registries that collect the data on adverse birth outcomes for surveillance purposes.

Several designs have been used in epidemologic studies of drinking water. Ecologic study designs are often used as screening tools in large populations. These studies are sometimes followed by case-control studies performed in the same population. In cohort or cross-sectional studies approaches, investigators compare disease rates of exposed and unexposed groups of residents living in an area with a particular water source or contaminant.

An advantage of the cohort and cross-sectional approach is that it allows the investigators to analyze data on multiple outcomes. This type of study might simultaneously examine the effect of water contaminants on birth defects, birth weight, gestational age at birth, and spontaneous abortions. However, in studies of specific contamination events, the small size of the populations limits the study's ability to detect moderate effects (e.g., risk (rate) ratios of 3.0 or more) for such a rare outcome as birth defects.

Studies using registries of a specific malformation can overcome these limitations by providing a large number of cases that are identified over time or for a larger geographic area. Case-control studies drawing on a single registry for a particular defect, however, are by definition limited to studying a single outcome. Ecologic study designs allow the combination of information from birth records and birth defect registries for large populations and over long periods. Ecologic studies, however, are prone to biases not encountered in individual level studies and, thus, are considered more limited with respect to causal inferences than are cohort or case-control studies.

The main methodological limitation of many epidemiologic studies of drinking water contaminants, independent of the design employed, stems from retrospective assessment of exposure. Interviews with study subjects or historical records designed for other purposes are the usual source of such information. The chemicals measured routinely at one location in the community might not reflect the composition of the drinking water in the home of a pregnant woman or the levels of contaminants in the water at the time of embryonic development. Another problem, known as recall bias, is introduced when exposure data (amount of tap water use) is collected retrospectively in interviews from women having infants with and without an adverse outcome. Interview information has proven extremely vulnerable to recall bias in situations of heightened public awareness of an environmental problem. For example, Fenster et al. (1992) concluded that the results from earlier studies linking contaminated tap water use to spontaneous abortions in Santa Clara County may be attributable to recall bias: Women who suffered a spontaneous abortion were aware of the water contamination problem and, thus, were more prone to report tap water use during pregnancy.

The published epidemiologic studies of drinking water and adverse birth outcomes are summarized in Table A.1 in Appendix A. The table summarizes the methods and results of these studies. Within this table, the studies are listed alphabetically by author.

In the following sections, selected results related to each outcome are discussed using information from these tables.

Studies of Drinking Water Contaminants and Spontaneous Abortions

Increased rates of spontaneous abortions have been associated with increased levels of mercury, arsenic, potassium, and silica in drinking water and with surface water as a source (Aschengrau et al., 1989). In Santa Clara County, an incident of well contamination with organic solvents from an industrial complex was associated with an increased risk of spontaneous abortions (Deane et al., 1989). This result was not confirmed in another area receiving contaminated water (Wrensch et al., 1992) and may be attributable to recall bias among women who had experienced a spontaneous abortion in the contaminated water area (Fenster et al., 1992). Lagakos et al. (1986) found no association between spontaneous abortion and exposure to chemical contaminants in the drinking water in Woburn, Massachusetts. Savitz et al. (1995) were unable to find a consistent relationship between water source and THM concentration and medically treated cases of miscarriage. The one possible exception was an increased risk of miscarriage in the highest sextile of THM concentration (adjusted odds ratio (OR) = 2.8, 95 percent confidence interval (CI) = 1.1–2.7) in Orange and Durham counties, North Carolina.

Two recently published studies have reexamined the association between drinking water and spontaneous abortion. A study of pregnant women in three California counties measured the association between the amount and type of drinking water consumed at 8 weeks' gestation and the spontaneous abortion rate (Swan et al., 1998). In one of the three counties in the study, consuming a high volume of cold tap water (six or more glasses per day) compared to none was associated with an elevated spontaneous abortion rate (OR = 2.17, 95% CI = 1.22–3.87) confirming earlier studies (Windham et al., 1992; Hertz-Picciotto et al., 1992; Wrensch et al., 1992). An even stronger association was observed between those consuming a high volume of cold tap water and no bottled water compared with those consuming high amounts of bottled water and no cold tap water (OR = 4.58, 95% CI = 1.97–10.64). Another study of the same population examined the relation between total and each of four THMs in drinking water (chloroform, bromoform, bromodichloromethane, and chlorodibromomethane), water consumption, and spontaneous abortions (Waller et al., 1998). High total THMs (TTHMs) and particularly high bromodichloromethane exposure was associated with a higher spontaneous abortion rate in a model that included other THM levels (OR = 3.0, 95% CI = 1.4–6.6) and in a model that did not (OR = 2.0; 95% CI = 1.2–3.5) in all three study areas.

Studies of Drinking Water and Low Birth Weight and Preterm Delivery

Few studies have examined the association between water contaminants and low birth weight. Intrauterine growth retardation has been associated with increased chloroform concentrations in drinking water in Iowa (Kramer et al., 1992). Bove et al. (1995) also described an association between TTHM and carbon tetrachloride and the health outcomes "small for gestational age" and "lower birth weight" in a New Jersey population. TTHM and carbon tetrachloride were associated with higher rates of being born "small for gestational age." At levels of 100 ppb, TTHM was also associated with lower birth weight, with an average difference of 70.4 grams among full-term births. Carbon tetrachloride was also associated with an increased rate of low and very low birth weight infants. Savitz et al. (1995) used data from a case-control study of miscarriage, preterm delivery, and low birth weight in central North Carolina to evaluate risk associated with water source, amount, and THM concentration. Neither water source nor THM level in the study was associated with increased rates of low birth weight. Given the limited quality of the exposure assessment, however, the authors recommended further research using more refined exposure measures.

Studies of Drinking Water and Birth Defects

Central nervous system (CNS) defects and the occurrence of anencephalus have been associated with water hardness (soft water increasing the risk) (Lowe et al., 1971), industrial contamination of drinking water wells with organic solvents (trichloroethylene, tetrachloroethylene, and chloroform) (Lagakos et al., 1986; Bove et al., 1995), and increased levels of nitrate in drinking water (Dorsch et al., 1984). Another study, however, did not find an association between water source (groundwater versus surface water) or drinking water treatment (chlorination versus chloramination) and the occurrence of birth defects (Aschengrau et al., 1989).

Numerous early correlation studies failed to yield consistent or conclusive findings regarding an association between trace elements in drinking water and neural tube defects (Penrose, 1957; Fedrick, 1970; Fielding and Smithells, 1971; Lowe et al., 1971; Morton et al., 1976; Bound et al., 1981). Later studies have reported mixed results. One found no association between drinking water trace elements and anencephalus (Elwood and Coldman, 1981). Another found an association between cardiovascular defects and lead, CNS defects and potassium, and ear, face, and neck defects and detectable silver levels (Aschengrau et al., 1993). Cohn et al. (1994) found an association between drinking water containing THMs and chlorinated solvents and neural tube defects and oral clefts. However, the authors advise caution and state that the positive associations do not provide sufficient evidence to claim that these contaminants cause adverse reproductive outcomes at levels commonly found in drinking water systems.

A case-control study found an association between detectable levels of arsenic, mercury, and lead in drinking water and specific cardiac defects and between selenium and all birth defects combined (Zierler et al., 1988). An Australian case-control study (Dorsch et al., 1984) found an association between high nitrate content in wells supplying drinking water and residences in which mothers of children born with CNS and musculoskeletal defects lived during the first trimester. Deane et al. (1989) reported increased risk for 14 birth defects combined in an area with contamination of the drinking water by an industrial solvent leak. Swan et al. (1989) extended the study to include a larger geographic area served by the contaminated wells and a longer time period to be able to investigate a subgroup of cardiac defects. Although a twofold increased risk for major cardiac defects was observed in the exposed area during the period of water contamination compared to the unexposed areas and the same area during periods of no water contamination, the occurrence of the cases in time and space was considered inconsistent with the contamination episode. In another study in Santa Clara County, Shaw et al. (1990) observed an association between cardiac defects and consumption of more than four glasses of tap water per day during the first trimester of pregnancy. A study by Goldberg et al. (1990) found an elevated rate of congenital heart defects among births to women residing in census tracts served with water contaminated by trichloroethylene during the first trimester of pregnancy. A recently completed case-control study found an association between neural tube defects and THMs, and between chlorine residuals and neural tube defects (Klotz et al., 1999).

SUMMARY

Over the last few decades, many epidemiologic studies have measured the association between contaminants in drinking water and adverse birth outcomes, including spontaneous abortions, birth defects, low birth weight, and preterm births. The plausibility of external factors affecting the development of a human fetus has been established with the identification of numerous human teratogens. In addition, many maternal characteristics have been associated with increased risk of impaired prenatal development. Although no conclusive evidence currently exists regarding an etiologic role of drinking water contaminants in the development of these outcomes, many studies have reported associations. This suggestive evidence provides the rationale for conducting a study of the association between reclaimed water and adverse birth outcomes.

Several studies have investigated the relationship between drinking water and spontaneous abortions, low birth weight, and birth defects.[1] From the spontaneous abortion studies, the most consistent finding is an association between high tap water consumption and the risk of spontaneous abortion. Results on the association between low birth weight/preterm delivery and exposure to drinking water contaminants have been mixed, with some indicating higher risk and others showing no association. Studies of birth defects have yielded a possible association between cardiac defects and industrial contamination of drinking water and high tap water consumption and between neural tube defects and disinfection by-products in drinking water.

---

[1]Although spontaneous abortions could not be included in this study, they are of interest as outcomes because they are considered a measure of abnormal fetal development.

Chapter Three

METHODS

Since 1962, reclaimed water has been used to recharge the groundwater basin in the Montebello Forebay region of eastern Los Angeles County. During the 1960s, the domestic water supplies of this area contained a uniformly low percentage of reclaimed water. Between 1970 and 1993, the percentage of reclaimed water remained low in some water systems, whereas other water systems experienced a gradual but steady increase in the percentage of reclaimed water, reaching a maximum of 38 percent in some systems.

Using a cohort study design with a ZIP-code-level measure of exposure, this epidemiologic study examined the association between residence in areas being served different percentages of reclaimed water and several adverse birth outcomes. Existing data on births (1982–1993), infant deaths (1982–1993), and birth defects (1990–1993) were analyzed. Rates of the adverse birth outcomes were compared between the area in eastern Los Angeles County receiving reclaimed water and a matched control area in Los Angeles County not receiving any reclaimed water. Each birth was allocated to one of five exposure groups based on the average annual percentage of reclaimed water in the ZIP code. Logistic regression methods were used to generate odds ratios and confidence intervals to compare outcomes in the reclaimed water and control groups.

The rest of this chapter provides a detailed description of the methods, including data sources, definition of the adverse birth outcomes, estimation of exposure to reclaimed water, selection of control area, and statistical methods.

DATA SOURCES

Information on the birth outcomes (birth weight, gestational age, and birth defects) came from existing data collected on a routine and ongoing basis in Los Angeles County by public health agencies. The error rate in the data collection process, therefore, should not differ between the reclaimed water groups and the control group. Thus, the quality of the data is probably similar across all study groups.

Birth and Death Certificates

All singleton births to residents of the ZIP codes in the reclaimed water and control areas during the twelve-year period from 1982 through 1993 were included in the analysis of birth weight, gestational age, and infant mortality. These data were derived from the California Birth Cohort files obtained from the State of California Department of Health Services (DHS). These files contain records of all live births occurring among mothers who are residents of California. The death records of infants who die within the first year of life are matched and linked to their respective live birth records in the Birth Cohort file. The information on births and deaths in these files originates from birth and death certificates, respectively, recorded as part of the registration system for vital events. Each record contains a ZIP code based on the residential address of the mother at the time of birth.[1] The ZIP code allows the birth data to be linked with the exposure and population data.

California Birth Defects Monitoring Program

Data were obtained from the California Birth Defects Monitoring Program (CBDMP) for every birth defect occurring among infants born between July 1990 and December 1993 to residents of the reclaimed water and control areas. When this study was conducted, data on birth defects in Los Angeles County were available only for this period.[2] Birth defects are identified through the CBDMP, a public health program jointly operated by the DHS and the March of Dimes Birth Defects Foundation. The CBDMP identifies infants born with malformations, as well as malformed fetuses of 20 weeks or more gestation. This program has developed and analyzed a database that registers children with structural defects, chromosome anomalies, and syndromes. The registry does not include metabolic or inherited diseases; functional problems, such as mental retardation; or other abnormal pregnancy outcomes, such as low birth weight (Stierman, 1994).

The CBDMP registry uses active surveillance methods to identify fetuses and infants with birth defects up to one year of age (Croen et al., 1991).[3] Because hospitals and health care providers are not required to report children with birth defects to any centralized registry, active surveillance is the only method for complete ascertainment. CBDMP staff review hospital logs, the hospital discharge diagnosis index, birth certificates, and death certificates in order to identify all possible cases of birth defects. They then review the medical records for the children identified from these sources and abstract the information for inclusion in the registry. The registry currently contains data on more than 200 types of defects (Croen et al., 1991).

Cases must meet several criteria in order to be entered in the CBDMP registry (Hexter et al., 1990). First, only conditions diagnosed or treated in a hospital or by a geneticist are included in the database. Next, only those diagnoses written in the medical

---

[1]ZIP codes were used as the geographic link between the birth outcome data and the exposure data, because census tracts were not coded on the birth certificates for Los Angeles County for the years of this study.

[2]Los Angeles County births were first included in the CBDMP in July 1990. All Los Angeles County births and hospital admissions of infants under one year of age reviewed by the registry staff between mid-1990 and December 1993 were included in this study.

[3]Approximately 95 percent of structural birth defects are recognized by a child's first birthday (Stierman, 1994).

record are entered. There are no restrictions on the number of diagnoses recorded for any child and if a child visits more than one hospital, reports from each source are maintained at the registry as separate records. Finally, conditions considered "minor," which might have extremely varied clinical definitions, are excluded from the registry when present in isolation but are included if they are present when other birth defects are identified in the same child.

1990 Census

Data on the number and characteristics of person living in the reclaimed water and control areas were derived from the 1990 Census of Population and housing machine-readable files for California (Census of Population and Housing, 1991a, 1991b, 1991c). The count of persons by age and sex was derived from data from the Summary Tape File 1 (Census of Population and Housing, 1991a). The count of persons by age, sex, race/ethnicity was derived from data from the Summary Tape File 2 (Census of Population and Housing, 1991b). The demographic and socioeconomic characteristics used to describe the population living in the reclaimed water and control areas were calculated on the basis of data from the Summary Tape File 3 (Census of Population and Housing, 1991c).

DEFINITIONS OF ADVERSE BIRTH OUTCOMES

We examined a large number of biologically plausible adverse birth outcomes in this study. No biologic agents and only trace levels of a small number of chemical compounds have been found in groundwater recharged with reclaimed water in the Montebello Forebay (Nellor et al., 1984). We thus analyzed many adverse birth outcomes, rather than limiting the study to outcomes known to be, or suspected of being, caused by exposure to a specific chemical. Outcomes were classified into 24 categories—infant mortality, four related to prenatal development, and 19 for various types of birth defects.

Prenatal Development and Infant Mortality

The adverse birth outcomes related to prenatal development are defined as follows:

- Low birth weight among full-term births: a liveborn infant weighing less than 2,500 grams at the time of birth, restricted to births between 37 and 41 weeks of gestation (Bove et al. 1995), inclusive[4]

- Low birth weight among all births: a liveborn infant weighing less than 2,500 grams at the time of birth, restricted to births between 20 and 50 weeks of gestation (Bove et al. 1995), inclusive

- Preterm birth: a liveborn infant born at less than 37 weeks of gestation

---

[4]"Weeks of gestation" is defined as the length of pregnancy measured in weeks, calculated from the date of last menses and the birth date recorded on the birth certificate. These dates are not necessarily reported or recorded accurately.

- Very low birth weight among all births: a liveborn infant weighing less than 1,500 grams at the time of birth, restricted to births between 20 and 50 weeks of gestation, inclusive

- Infant mortality: a liveborn infant who dies within the first year of life (excluding deaths due to accidents and injuries).

The analyses of these outcomes address the important question of possible adverse effects of environmental toxicants on development of the fetus during gestation. Such an effect might manifest itself as intrauterine growth retardation resulting in birth weights below normal (low birth weight or very low birth weight) among full-term births or among all births (i.e., occurring at any gestational age). Because the gestational period might be shortened by the disruptive effects of an environmental toxin, we also analyzed the percentage of births occurring before full term (preterm births). Infant mortality was studied to allow comparison with the earlier studies of the Montebello Forebay, which also investigated patterns of infant mortality. Prenatal environmental exposures might be expected to influence infant mortality indirectly, if such exposure results in increased risk of birth defects or impaired development.

The study population for the analysis of these five outcomes consisted of 466,743 live births, identified from birth certificates, that occurred during the 12-year period (January 1, 1982, through December 31, 1993) among residents of 36 ZIP codes in Los Angeles County, California (for a list of all 36 ZIP codes, see Table 3.1). Multiple births were excluded from the analyses because of their higher risk of the outcomes related to prenatal development.

Birth Defects

Every birth defect identified in a liveborn infant during the first year of life was included in the analyses. Birth defects were divided into 19 categories, which were selected in consultation with the CBDMP. Some categories of defects were chosen for evaluation because they are among the most frequent and recognizable birth defects. As such, their reporting and documentation in the registry are useful for tracking time trends and surveillance purposes. These defects, called "sentinel defects" by the CBDMP, include oral clefts, pyloric stenosis, neural tube defects, limb defects, and intestinal atresias. In addition, patent ductus arteriosus was evaluated as a separate class of heart defects because of its strong association with preterm birth. The remaining birth defects were stratified based on the body systems in which they occurred. Each defect was assigned to an analytic category using the British Paediatric Association (BPA) code on the CBDMP record. The range of BPA codes in each category is shown in Table 3.2. Infants with defects classified as syndromes were analyzed separately. The syndrome defects were further categorized into "chromosomal syndromes" and "other syndromes" to distinguish between genetically based syndromes that are unlikely to be associated with environmental exposures and other syndromes.

Table 3.1

**ZIP Codes in Study Areas Used in the Analysis of
Adverse Birth Outcomes**

Montebello Forebay	Northeast San Fernando Valley
90022	91342
90023	91343
90040	91344
90063	91345
90201	91352
90240	91401
90241	91402
90242	91405
90262	91406
90280	91605
90602	91606
90603	
90604	Pomona
90605	91766
90606	91767
90631	91768
90640	
90650	
90660	
90670	
90706	
90723	

The study population for the analysis of birth defects consisted of 161,104 live births, identified using birth certificates, that occurred during a 3.5-year period (July 1, 1990 through December 31, 1993) among residents of 36 ZIP codes in Los Angeles County, California. Of these, 3,311 infants were identified as having a birth defect diagnosed within the first year of life by the CBDMP. Multiple births were also excluded from these analyses because of their higher risk of birth defects.

EXPOSURE TO RECLAIMED WATER

In the absence of information on individual consumption of tap water and specific organic compounds in reclaimed water, this study uses the percentage of reclaimed water in the ZIP code of residence as a surrogate measure of exposure to reclaimed water. Most organic compounds found in municipal wastewater cannot be identified at the molecular level because reliable techniques for detection and quantification do not exist (NRC, 1998). Also, complete toxicologic data are not available for the wide range of organic compounds found in wastewater. Thus, even if the organic fraction in reclaimed water could be analyzed completely, toxicologic data on the health risks associated with them would not be available. In the foreseeable future, therefore, the uncertainty regarding which compounds are present in reclaimed water and what health risks are associated with those compounds will persist.[5]

---

[5]This situation applies to municipal drinking water supplies in general, not just reclaimed wastewater.

Table 3.2

Categories of Birth Defects Used in Study

Birth Defect	BPA Code[a]
All defects	
Neural tube defects	740.000–741.999
Other nervous system	742.000–742.999
Ears, eyes, face, neck	743.000–744.999
Heart defects	745.000–745.499, 745.510– 746.999, 747.100–747.499
Patent ductus arteriosus	747.000
Other heart	745.500–745.509, 747.500– 747.900
Respiratory system	748.000–748.999
Cleft defects	749.000–749.999
Pyloric stenosis	750.510–750.519
Intestinal atresias	751.100–751.299
Other digestive	750.000–750.509, 750.520– 751.099, 751.300–751.999
Urogenital system	752.000–753.999
Limb defects	755.200–755.399
Other musculoskeletal	754.000–755.199, 755.400– 756.999
Integument	757.000–757.999
All other defects	759.000–759.999
Syndromes	
Chromosomal	758.000–758.999
Other	Selected codes, 740–759

[a]Birth defects were identified in the data using British Paediatric Association codes (British Paediatric Association, 1979).

The remainder of this section describes the methods used to calculate the percentage of reclaimed water for the water systems in the Montebello Forebay.

Estimating the Percentage of Reclaimed Water in Domestic Supplies

Estimating the percentage of reclaimed water in the water supplies of the Montebello Forebay was a critical first step in this research. Because reclaimed water cannot be labeled and traced through the system, the percentage of reclaimed water in household supplies must be estimated indirectly. The indirect estimation method was based on three parameters: the volume of reclaimed water used to recharge the groundwater basin; the design and location of a well, which influences how reclaimed water replaces groundwater; and the relative percentages of groundwater and surface water supplied to consumers by the water system. (See Appendix B for a detailed description of the methods.)

The volume of reclaimed water used to recharge the groundwater basin is the primary determinant of the percentage of reclaimed water in the groundwater pumped out of the Montebello Forebay of the Central Basin. Over the past 40 years, several sources of water have been used to recharge the groundwater basin, including imported surface supplies (the State Water Project Aqueduct conveying supplies from Northern California and the Colorado River Aqueduct providing water from the Colorado River), as well as storm runoff and reclaimed water. During the 1950s, the groundwater basin was recharged with water imported from the Colorado River and local storm runoff. In the early 1960s, groundwater recharge with reclaimed water began and recharge with other sources continued. In the mid-1970s, the volume of Colorado River water used for recharge diminished and was replaced with State Water Project supplies imported by the Metropolitan Water District of Southern California (MWD). Since then, the relative and absolute volumes of reclaimed water used to recharge the Montebello Forebay groundwater basin have increased. Therefore, it can be assumed that the proportion of reclaimed water delivered to consumers in the Montebello Forebay has also increased substantially.

The percentage of reclaimed water in a particular water supply in the Montebello Forebay also depends on the design and location of the well. In general, it takes less time for recharge water to reach wells closer to the spreading grounds than to reach wells farther away. The rate and direction of flow in the groundwater basin is also affected by factors other than distance, including basin geology, soil permeability, pumping rates, and basin hydraulic gradients (which reflect relative basin water levels). To account for this, the analysis incorporated data on the time it takes for recharge water to reach a well, based on well water quality samples from locations throughout the basin rather than only on the distance between the well and the spreading grounds. This measure is referred to in this report as the "replacement lag time."

The relative amounts of surface water and groundwater used by a single water system can fluctuate significantly from year to year and even from season to season. A mixture of groundwater and surface water supplies the residential, business, and industrial customers of water systems of the Montebello Forebay. Water systems personnel make decisions regarding the use of these two sources on the basis of availability and cost. Data on which water sources were used and how much of each source was used (production levels for individual wells) were incorporated into the estimates of the reclaimed water.

Estimating the percentage of reclaimed water supplied to residential customers in the Montebello Forebay consisted of several steps. Data on the three factors discussed above—the volume of reclaimed water used in the recharge process, the replacement lag time for wells throughout the Montebello Forebay, and the relative amounts of groundwater and surface water used by each water system—were collected from regional water agencies and individual water systems. These data were then used in calculating the percentage of reclaimed water. The data collection and analysis were conducted by Bookman-Edmonston Engineering, Inc., an engineering firm specializing in water resources.

The current study extends the geographic area and the period beyond those used in the Sloss et al. (1996) study. Percentages of reclaimed water for the additional water system service areas and time, therefore, had to be calculated by Bookman-Edmonston Engineering, Inc. The report documenting the results of these calculations provides annual estimates of the percentage of reclaimed water for each water service area in the Montebello Forebay, including revised estimates of some data used in the earlier study (Bookman-Edmonston Engineering, Inc., 1998). The remainder of this section summarizes the methods and findings used by Bookman-Edmonston Engineering, Inc., in these calculations.

Identifying Water Purveyors in the Montebello Forebay

The geographic area included in the current study differs slightly from that used in the earlier study (Sloss et al., 1996). In the current study, we used ZIP codes as the geographic unit to link the health and exposure data, whereas census tracts were used earlier. Because of this difference, decisions related to which areas should be included had to be reevaluated. Eleven water systems were added because of revised study boundaries formed by the ZIP codes. The current study includes a total of 38 water systems (Table 3.3).

Several water systems in the Montebello Forebay contain more than one service area. Each service area was treated separately in calculating the percentage of reclaimed water, because the operating parameters differ by service area, not by water system. There are 92 service areas contained within the aforementioned 38 water systems.

Data on the operating practices were collected for the 36-year period from 1960–1995 by Bookman-Edmonston Engineering, Inc., for all Montebello Forebay water systems used in the Sloss et al. (1996) study. For the water systems added for the current study, Bookman-Edmonston Engineering, Inc., collected data only for the years 1977–1995. The information requested from each water system service area included the boundaries of its service areas, the number of residential connections, the sources of water used, and the production levels for each well within a service area. The staff at Bookman-Edmonston Engineering, Inc., used this information in determining the percentage of reclaimed water in the systems' supplies (Bookman-Edmonston, Engineering, Inc., 1993, 1998).

Estimating the Percentage of Reclaimed Water in Groundwater Supplies

The first step in estimating the percentage of reclaimed water in household water supplies was to estimate the percentage of reclaimed water in the groundwater supply used by each water system service area. For each service area, the percentage of reclaimed water in the groundwater supply was calculated for each year between 1977 and 1995.[6] One or more of four statistical techniques were employed in estimating the percentage of reclaimed water in the groundwater supply. They were (1) direct calculation from a sulfate ion model (Nellor et al., 1984), (2) regression analysis (Weisberg, 1985), (3) the Kriging analytic method (Davis and McCullaugh, 1975), and (4) an analysis of travel time contours (similar to the sulfate ion model described in

---

[6]Percentages for 1960–1976 were based on calculations performed as part of the Health Effects Study by the Los Angeles County Sanitation Districts and Bookman-Edmonston Engineering, Inc. (Nellor et al., 1984).

Table 3.3

**Montebello Forebay Water Systems Included and
Excluded from Epidemiologic Assessment**

Systems Included in Study	Map No.[a]	Systems Excluded from Study	Map No.[a]
Bellflower-Somerset Mutual Water	33	City of Compton	38
California Water Service Company	1	La Hacienda Water Company	40
City of Downey	3	Los Angeles County Water Works No. 10	41
City of Huntington Park	34	Lynwood Park Mutual Water Company	42
La Habra Heights County Water District	6	Midland Park Water Trust	45
City of Lynwood	24		
Maywood Mutual Water Co. No. 3	25		
City of Montebello	8		
Montebello Land and Water Company	9		
Mutual Water Owners Assoc., Los Nietos	7		
City of Norwalk	10		
Orchard Dale County Water District	11		
City of Paramount	35		
Park Water Company	12		
Peerless Land and Water Company	26		
Pico County Water District	13		
City of Pico Rivera	14		
Rancho Los Amigos	28		
San Gabriel Valley Water Company	15		
City of Santa Fe Springs	16		
City of South Gate	30		
South Montebello Irrigation District	17		
Southern California Water Company	18		
Southwest Suburban Water Company	19		
Tract No. 180 Mutual Water Co.	31		
Tract No. 349 Mutual Water Co.	32		
City of Whittier	20		
Bellflower Home Garden	36		
Bigby Townsite	37		
City of Commerce	5		
County Water Co.	39		
Maywood No. 1	43		
Maywood No. 2	44		
Walnut Park Mutual Water Company	46		
Beverly Acres Mutual Water Users Association	47		
Industry Water Works	48		
Los Angeles Department of Water and Power	49		
City of Vernon	50		

[a]Numbers refer to map of Montebello Forebay water system service areas (available on request).

Nellor et al., 1984).[7] These methods are described in detail in Appendix B. Multiple methods were required because some techniques could not be used with the data available. In general, the sulfate ion model could be used as a "stand-alone" technique only for data from 1977 through 1982. Regression analysis was used for the subset of data between 1983 and 1995 that exhibited a correlation of 0.80 or

[7]Methods 2 through 4 were based on the sulfate ion model with the addition of other techniques to modify the results.

greater between the results of this method and the sulfate ion model. The Kriging technique was used for 1983–1995 data with correlations lower than 0.80. The travel time contour method was used instead of the Kriging method for service areas in which no comparison wells were available. Using these four methods (described in more detail in Appendix B), Bookman-Edmonston Engineering, Inc., generated estimates of the percentage of reclaimed water in the groundwater pumped by each water system service area in the Montebello Forebay (Bookman-Edmonston, Inc., 1993, 1998).

Estimating Reclaimed Water Percentages by Service Area

The final step in estimating reclaimed water percentages incorporates information on how much groundwater is pumped by each water system. Because only pumped groundwater (not surface water) contains reclaimed water, the percentage of reclaimed water served in any given year depends on the percentage of groundwater pumped by the water system during that year. For each water system, the average annual percentage of groundwater in the total volume of water served was estimated by the staff at Bookman-Edmonston Engineering, Inc., using operations data obtained from the water systems. This information was used to calculate the annual percentage of reclaimed water in the total supply for each water system service area, as follows:

$$T_{rw} = T_{gw} \times G_{rw} ,$$

where T_{rw} = percentage of reclaimed water in total supply

T_{gw} = percentage of pumped groundwater in total supply

G_{rw} = percentage of reclaimed water in pumped groundwater.

The percentage of reclaimed water in the total supply was calculated for each water year[8] between 1977 and 1995 for each of the 92 water system service areas. These percentages served as the basis for classifying the births into exposure groups for the statistical analysis of the birth outcomes. (These data are reproduced in Appendix B.)

Of the 92 service areas, 58 served some percentage of reclaimed water at some time during the 19-year period, 1977–1995. The maximum annual percentage of reclaimed water in the water supplies served by the 58 water systems varied greatly, from less than 1 percent to 38 percent.

LINKING EXPOSURE DATA WITH OTHER DATA

ZIP code areas were the geographic unit used to link data on reclaimed water exposure with the health outcome data in the study. To do this, we compared the bound-

---

[8]A water year is the period October 1 through September 30.

aries of the water system service areas and ZIP codes on a street map of the Montebello Forebay region. We identified 22 ZIP codes that overlapped the 58 Montebello Forebay service areas that had served reclaimed water sometime during the study period of 1982 through 1993. In many cases, the boundaries of the service areas and the ZIP codes did not match, and ZIP codes were split between two or more water systems. The percentage of reclaimed water for each ZIP code was calculated as the weighted average of the percentages of reclaimed water served in the service areas within the ZIP code boundaries.

We estimated the percentage of reclaimed water at the ZIP-code level using the estimated proportion of the births in the ZIP code that occurred within the service area as a weighting factor. Within some ZIP codes, the population and the number of births are not distributed uniformly. Therefore, in calculating the weighted average of reclaimed water served in a ZIP code, using the service areas' proportion of the births rather than the proportion of the geographic area in the ZIP code as a weighting factor might more accurately reflect the average "exposure to reclaimed water" of pregnant women in the ZIP code. Because we do not know the mother's actual address, we are unable to estimate directly the distribution of births within the ZIP code. For three years within the study period (1982–1984), we have information on the number of births by census tract. Because census tracts are smaller, more homogeneous units, we assume that households with births are uniformly distributed within the census tract. Therefore, we assumed the proportion of births in the intersection of a service area and a census tract (B_{stz}) is equal to the proportion of the area in the intersection of a service area and a census tract, that is, $B_{stz} = B_{tz}(A_{stz}/A_{tz})$. We pooled the number of births from 1982 to 1984 to reduce the variability by census tract by year.

We used the following procedure to estimate the number of births for each water system service area within a given ZIP code. For any given ZIP code z and service area s that intersects that ZIP code, we define the estimated number of births, B_{sz} by the following:

$$B_{sz} = \sum_t B_{stz} = \sum_t B_{tz} A_{stz} / A_{tz}, \ A_{tz} = \sum_t A_{stz}$$

where B_{tz} denotes the number of births in the years 1982 to 1984 from households in census tract t[9] and ZIP z, A_{stz} denotes area in square meters of the intersection between service area s, census tract t, and ZIP code z. Summation is over all census tracts that cover the intersection of the service area and the ZIP code area.

Given the number of births for the service areas, the B_{sz}s, we estimate the percentage of reclaimed water served in the ZIP code by:

$$AP_{zy} = \sum_s P_{sy} B_{sz} / B_z, \ B_z = \sum_s B_{sz}$$

---

[9]The number of births by census tract was available for the three-year period from 1982 to 1984, but not available for births after 1984.

where AP_{zy} denotes the weighted average for the percentage of reclaimed water served in ZIP code area z in year y, P_{sy} denotes the percentage of reclaimed water served in service area s in year y, and B_z denotes the number of births in ZIP code z. Summation is over all service areas that intersect the ZIP code area.

The percentage of reclaimed water (i.e., the weighted average of water supplies within the ZIP code) is assigned to each birth record, using the ZIP code of the mother's residence at the time of birth. The statistical models used in the analysis are fit to individual birth records, not to aggregated data from each ZIP code. Therefore, we must assign an exposure to each birth. As mentioned above, the percentage of reclaimed water in the mother's tap water would be the best measure of exposure to reclaimed water. However, this measure is not available. Because the mother's ZIP code is known only for a single point in time (i.e., the time of birth), we are able to estimate the percentage of reclaimed water in the mother's drinking water only around the time of birth and not for the entire pregnancy. The measure of exposure in the statistical models is the percentage of reclaimed water served to the ZIP code area in the year that an infant was born. Even if we assume that movement across ZIP code areas is roughly constant over a year and that moving from a lower percentage ZIP code to a higher percentage ZIP code is about as likely as moving from a higher percentage ZIP code to a lower percentage ZIP code, some births may be misclassified with regard to exposure and the estimated odds ratios might be lower than the true value.

In the statistical analyses, each birth was assigned to one of five groups based on the percentage of reclaimed water served to the ZIP code of the mother's residence during the year of birth. The five groups are defined as follows:

- control: 0 percent
- RW 1: more than 0 to less than 2 percent
- RW 2: from 2 to less than 5 percent
- RW 3: from 5 to less than 15 percent
- RW 4: 15 percent and higher.

We decided on the number of groups (five) and the cutpoints defining the groups based on the following: being able to compare rates among several groups of births with increasing exposure to reclaimed water, having an approximately equal number of births in each of the reclaimed water groups, and following natural breaks in the percentage of reclaimed water.

SELECTION OF CONTROL AREA

Selection of the control area was aimed at identifying an area in Los Angeles County that did not receive any reclaimed water but otherwise had characteristics mirroring the reclaimed water areas. The control area in the current study was chosen during the earlier study of cancer, mortality, and infectious disease.[10]   Matching the characteristics of the populations living in the control area with the characteristics of those living in the exposed areas minimizes the effects of possible confounders[11] on the results.   By matching the reclaimed water and control areas on confounding variables that may be important in determining rates of the adverse birth outcomes, observed differences will more likely be attributable to reclaimed water than to the other confounding variables.   Matching the characteristics of the populations living in the control areas with the characteristics of those living in the reclaimed water areas has the added benefit of increasing the statistical power of the analysis (i.e., the probability that we will detect a difference when in fact a difference exists).   Profiles for several possible control areas were developed, containing information on population characteristics as well as variables related to the relevant water supplies.

After an extensive search, we identified two locations in Los Angeles County to use as a control area matched with the areas receiving reclaimed water.   These locations were chosen on the basis of demographic and socioeconomic characteristics similar to the Montebello Forebay, the lack of known volatile organic compound groundwater contamination, and the absence of reclaimed water.   Many possible control areas were eliminated because of groundwater contamination.   Some were a closer match demographically to the Montebello Forebay than were the control groups selected.   The ZIP codes in the control area are in the Pomona area of eastern Los Angeles County and in the northeastern San Fernando Valley in northern Los Angeles County (see Figure 3.1).

The Pomona control location includes three ZIP codes in the eastern area of Los Angeles County.   After the area was matched on the basis of population characteristics, the staff at Bookman-Edmonston Engineering, Inc., evaluated information from the City of Pomona on historical water quality in the area (Morgan, 1994a).   The water served to Pomona residents is derived from three sources: groundwater wells, supplies imported from outside the Los Angeles area by the Metropolitan Water District of Southern California, and surface supplies obtained from San Antonio Canyon.   Pomona water supplies have never contained reclaimed water.   The other control area consists of 11 ZIP codes in the northeastern San Fernando Valley.   Of these, 10 receive surface water only from the City of Los Angeles Department of Water and Power.   The remaining ZIP code is supplied by the City of San Fernando water system, with a mixture of groundwater and surface water.   These supplies have never contained reclaimed water and never been affected by groundwater contamination (Morgan, 1994b, 1994c).

---

[10]For further detail, see Sloss et al. (1996).

[11]A "confounder" is a factor that is a determinant (or cause) of the outcome and is unequally distributed among those exposed and those not exposed. Not controlling for a confounder in an analysis results in "confounding," which is a distortion of a true effect of an exposure on an outcome by its association with other factors that can influence the outcome (Last, 1983).

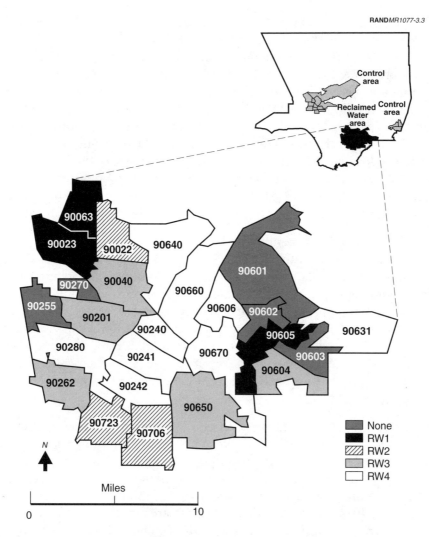

NOTE: Groups RW1 to RW4 shown are based on exposure data for 1991.

Figure 3.1—Montebello Forebay Region of Los Angeles County: ZIP Codes in
Exposure Groups Used in Analysis

STATISTICAL METHODS

The relationship between reclaimed water and the various birth outcomes was analyzed using multivariate logistic regression. Such models provide an estimate of the
ratios of the rates of adverse birth outcomes from populations receiving varying percentages of reclaimed water, while adjusting for other differences among the populations. Even after selecting a control population similar to the reclaimed water
population, differences in demographic and socioeconomic characteristics remain.
In addition, the characteristics of births differ among populations in the Montebello
Forebay that receive different levels of reclaimed water (Tables 4.2 and 4.3). To control for the possibly confounding effects of such differences, we include covariates in

the regression models that might affect the rate of adverse birth outcomes. The results of these analyses are presented in the tables throughout Chapter Four.

Logistic Regression Analysis of Birth Outcome Data

We modeled the occurrence of a birth outcome, such as a preterm birth, as a function of demographic and other variables and exposure to reclaimed water. We fit the models using individual birth outcomes. For the births in the reclaimed water and control areas, we fit a logistic regression model which estimates the underlying probability of an outcome, p, based on the observed binary data (1 if the outcome occurs, 0 otherwise). The basic form of the model is:

$$\log\left(\frac{p}{1-p}\right) = i + r_i + a_j + s_k + \ldots + e_l$$

where the log of the odds of an adverse birth outcome, $p/(1-p)$, are assumed to be linearly determined by the ith racial-ethnic group, of the jth mother's age group, of the kth child's gender, in the lth exposure group (and where the dots indicate that other covariates were used in various models). The covariates used in the various models are listed in Table 3.4. The intercept i corresponds to the overall log odds of a birth outcome across all groups and the other parameters denote the additive effect of being a member of a particular group.

Outcomes (Dependent Variables). As mentioned above, we fit separate models for each of the 24 adverse birth outcomes. For each observation, the dependent variable was coded as 1 if the adverse birth outcome occurred (e.g., low birth weight if the infant weighed less than 2,500 grams at birth), and 0 otherwise. For birth defects, we set the dependent variable equal to 1 if the infant had been identified as having a specific defect by the CBDMP (i.e., coded with specific BPA codes, as listed in Table 3.2) and 0 otherwise.

Covariates (Independent Variables). We selected model variables using two main criteria: scientific validity and statistical significance. Based on the first criterion of scientific validity, we included variables, such as race/ethnicity, that have been associated with these outcomes in previous epidemiologic studies. In some cases, the coefficients for such variables were not statistically significant in the models we tested. Based on the second criterion of statistical significance, we included variables for which the model coefficient was statistically significant, after carefully evaluating such significance in terms of findings from previous studies. Conversely, the variables we dropped from the models showed no statistical significance (in general, across our family of models) and had no known effect on the model outcome. The set of variables included in the birth defect and prenatal developmental models is different because of data availability. For example, mother's education was not available from birth certificates for the years 1982–1988 and therefore could not be used in the prenatal development models. Similarly, the inadequate prenatal care variable could not be calculated for 1982–1988 birth records, because it was based, in part, on the number of prenatal visits, another variable not available for those years. We included birth year in the birth defect models because of year-to-year variation in numbers of birth defects that might be attributable to events unrelated to reclaimed water (e.g., an outbreak of rubella).

We created categorical variables to represent each of the demographic, socio-economic, and health status characteristics included in the models. Such variables as race, inadequate prenatal care, and birthplace of mother are categorical variables by definition. For such variables as mother's age, we created categories based on the continuous variable.[12] Fixed effects for birth year were entered in the birth defects models to account for temporal changes, such as a known outbreak of rubella during the study period. The known inadequate care indicator was derived from information about the child's gestational age, the number of prenatal visits, and the month prenatal care began. It was defined as follows: If prenatal care began in the seventh month or later, regardless of the other variables, prenatal care was defined as inadequate. For all other records, known inadequate care was defined as a function of the child's gestational age and the number of prenatal visits. As the gestational age increased, the number of prenatal visits required to be adequate increased (Table 3.5). (We based this variable on the "three-factor health services index" described in Table 2-3 of Kessner et al. (1973) but redefined it based on which data elements were available.)

As described above, the inadequate prenatal care variable was derived from three other variables: weeks of gestation, number of prenatal visits, and month prenatal care began. Because one of these variables—number of prenatal visits—was not available for the years 1982–1988, we could not calculate the inadequate prenatal care variable for those years. Because of this, we also could not include this variable in the prenatal development models that utilized data for the years 1982–1993. Because the data necessary for calculating the inadequate care variable were available for the entire period of the birth defect analysis (i.e., 1990–1993), we were able to include them in the birth defect models. We tested the effect of the inadequate care variable in the prenatal development models for 1982–1988 and found that the study conclusions would not have been different from those reported here.

Parameter Estimation

To estimate the parameters of the models, we used maximum-likelihood methods. Maximum-likelihood estimates are the values of the parameters that make the

---

[12]The use of categorical variables allows for general nonlinearities in the relationship between age and outcome. To determine the cutpoints for the categorical variables, results from previously published studies of generalized additive models (GAMs) were used. GAMs fit a smooth, but not necessarily linear, relationship between age and outcomes. However, because GAMs are computer-intensive we could not use GAMs for fitting all the models and the full dataset. Instead, we used GAMs on random subsets of the data to determine first, the functional relationship between age and outcome, and then, appropriate cutpoints.

Table 3.4

Covariates Used in Logistic Regression Models

	Outcome	
	Prenatal Development and Infant Mortality[a]	Birth Defects
Mother's Race/Ethnicity		
White, African-American, Hispanic,[b] Asian, Other	X	X
Mother's Age[c]	X	X
Child's Gender		
Male, female[b]	X	X
Median Housing Value		
By ZIP code from the 1990 census	X	
Birthplace of Mother		
United States, Mexico, other[b]	X	
Birth Order		
First child, second or third child,[b] fourth or subsequent child	X	
Maternal Medical Problems		
Cardiac, kidney, neither[b]	X	
Weeks of Gestation		
Numeric	X	
Months Since Last Live Birth		
Numeric; coded 0 if firstborn	X	
Month Prenatal Care Began		
Numeric; coded 1–9 for each month, 10 if prenatal care was never provided	X	
Number Previous Infant Deaths		
Numeric	X	
Adequacy 0f Prenatal Care		
Known inadequate, other[b] (see Table 3.5 for definition)		X
Year of Birth		
1990, 1991, 1992,[b] 1993		X
Mother's Education		
Less than 9 years of school, 9 to 12 years,[b] more than 12 years		X
Exposure		
0,[b] more than 0 to <2%, 2–<5%, 5–<15%, 15% or higher	X	X

[a]Birth weight and infant mortality models also included interaction terms between age and the race category of African-American.

[b]Reference categories.

[c]Age categories used in birth weight models: Very young (less than 17 years), young (17–20),[b] middle (21–30), and older (older than 30). Categories used in birth defect models: young (less than 20), middle (20–34),[b] and older (35 or older).

observed outcomes most probable under the likelihood model. If the assumed model is a reasonable approximation to the process generating the data, maximum-likelihood estimates have certain desirable statistical properties.

The parameter estimates generated by the logistic regression model may be used to calculate the log odds of the probability of an outcome, given particular demographic and other covariates. The model can also be used to estimate the adjusted odds

Table 3.5

Definition of Known Inadequate Prenatal Care Variable

If prenatal care began after the seventh month, or					
if gestational age is between a and b (weeks), *and*	(a, b) (0, 21)	(22, 29)	(30, 31)	(32, 33)	(34, _)
number of prenatal visits is less than or equal to	0	1	2	3	4

ratios that compare the risk of the outcome of interest in a reclaimed water group and the control group. The adjusted odds ratio is calculated by exponentiating the exposure parameter for each of the reclaimed water groups, RW 1–RW 4.

Variability of Parameter Estimates

For any particular outcome, we estimated the model parameters based on the assumption that, conditional on the covariates in the model, the outcomes among individuals are uncorrelated. This assumption, however, might not be correct. In particular, the risk of an adverse birth outcome could be more similar for individuals living within the same ZIP code than for individuals living in different ZIP codes. For example, the model might miss important environmental exposures that are geographically distributed and, therefore, result in higher risks for individuals living in some ZIP codes than in others. Similarly, characteristics that might be more homogeneous within than between ZIP codes, but are not in the model, might result in risks within a ZIP code being more similar than risks in different ZIP codes. Ignoring such correlation can lead to inefficient estimation of parameters and underestimation of standard errors.

There are several methods for accounting for possible heterogeneity across ZIP codes, including hierarchical models (Breslow and Clayton, 1993) or generalized estimating equations (GEE) (Liang and Zeger, 1986; Prentice and Zhao, 1991). We chose to use the GEE approach of Liang and Zeger (1986) with a working independence matrix. This method requires fitting the maximum-likelihood estimates, assuming no heterogeneity, and then adjusting the standard errors to allow for possible violations of that assumption. The SUDAAN Software (Shah et al., 1987)[13] was used to estimate the standard errors. Compared to the estimates described in Liang and Zeger, this software adjusts the standard error estimates with a constant $(n-1)/n$ bias correction, where n is the number of ZIP codes in the data. For confidence intervals and hypothesis tests, we used a reference t-distribution with $(n-1)$ degrees of freedom rather than the standard normal distribution. Using a reference t-distribution yielded confidence intervals that are 3 percent wider than those based on the standard normal.

---

[13]For birth defects outcomes we used SAS macros written to replicate the SUDAAN routines.

Imputation, Missing Values, and Sample Sizes in Models

Most of the covariates listed in Table 3.4 had a small percentage of missing values, generally less than 1 percent of the total data set. In the data used in the analysis of prenatal development and infant mortality, covariates with a higher percentage of missing values were weeks of gestation (2.6 percent missing), months since last live birth (4 percent), and number of prenatal visits (5.2 percent). In the birth defect data, covariates with a higher percentage of missing values were month prenatal care began (1 percent) and the number of prenatal visits (1.7 percent).

Records missing either the dependent variable or one or more of the covariates were excluded from the analysis. To minimize the number of records that had to be excluded, we imputed values for records missing the number of prenatal visits and month prenatal care began by assigning the mean value by race-ethnicity within a ZIP code. For example, an Asian mother missing the number of prenatal visits was assigned the mean number of prenatal visits among all Asian mothers in her ZIP code.

Of 466,743 records available for the analysis of prenatal development outcomes, 14,468 (3.1 percent) were excluded from the analysis because gestational ages under 20 weeks or longer than 50 weeks are considered clinically implausible and thus in error. For the prenatal development models that included gestational age, 1.1 percent of 452,275 records were excluded for missing covariates after imputation, resulting in 447,028 records in the model. For the preterm birth models, 1.1 percent of records were excluded because of missing covariates, resulting in 447,248 records in the model. For the infant mortality models, 1.3 percent of the records were excluded because of missing data, resulting in 460,866 records in the model. For the low birth weight models based on full-term births only, 1.1 percent of records were excluded because of missing data, resulting in 330,438 records in the model.

The initial birth defects data set contained 161,104 records. For the analysis of syndrome defects (both chromosomal syndromes and other syndromes), we excluded 776 records (0.5 percent) from the models because of missing covariates. Therefore, 160,328 records remained for fitting the models for defect syndromes. For modeling birth defects other than syndromes, we excluded the 486 infants with defect syndromes. Thus, the initial data contained only 160,623 records. In addition, 773 (0.5 percent) records were missing values for one or more covariates and, therefore, were excluded from the model. Hence, a total of 159,850 records were used to fit these 17 birth defect models.

Because missing data could also occur in the dependent variable, the number of records in each analysis varies slightly. Observations with implausible values for gestational age were not excluded from the models for infant mortality or birth defects because the model did not include gestational age as a covariate. Inaccurate reporting of gestational age was not viewed as evidence of overall low data quality for a record. Table 3.6 shows the initial number of records, the number of records excluded because gestational age was less than 20 or greater than 50 weeks, the number of records excluded because of missing data in the dependent or independent variables, and the final number of records included in the model.

Sensitivity Analysis

To test the sensitivity of the estimated exposure effects to the model parameters, we repeated the analyses of the birth outcomes data with several alternative models. The sensitivity of the estimated effect of reclaimed water to the gestational age specification was evaluated by comparing model results for various subsets of the data. In particular, we constructed two models: one including all of the data, and the other including only births with gestational age between 20 and 50 weeks (inclusive). Births with gestational age less than 20 weeks and greater than 50 weeks are considered clinically implausible, so these birth records were considered incorrectly coded or otherwise in error. In general, the estimated effects of reclaimed water were insensitive to including births outside the range of 20 to 50 weeks gestation. Sensitivity to alternative restrictions on gestational age was tested for each birth outcome.

We also investigated the sensitivity of the results to including and excluding Pomona from the control group. Pomona was chosen during the Sloss et al. (1996) study as part of the control area. In a meeting of the Advisory Committee in 1998, it was suggested that Pomona may have had some level of groundwater contamination with perchlorate for some length of time during the study period. We repeated the analysis after removing births in the Pomona ZIP codes from the control group. The results from these models are discussed at the end of Chapter Four and presented in Appendixes E and F.

Table 3.6

Number of Records by Outcome: Initial, Excluded from Analysis, and Included in Analysis

Outcome	Initial	Number of Records				In Analysis	
		Excluded from Analysis					
		Weeks of Gestation Out-of-Range[a]		Missing Data			
Low birth weight with gestational age	466,743	14,468[a]	3.1%	5,247	1.1%	447,028	95.8%
Low birth weight	466,743	14,468[a]	3.1%	5,027	1.1%	447,248	95.8%
Low birth weight (full term only)	334,115			3,677	1.1%	330,438	98.9%
Very low birth weight	466,743	14,468[a]	3.1%	5,027	1.1%	447,028	95.8%
Preterm birth	466,743	14,468[a]	3.1%	5,027	1.1%	447,248	95.8%
Infant mortality	466,743	—	—	5,877	1.3%	460,866	98.7%
Birth defects other than syndromes	160,623	—	—	773	0.5%	159,850	99.5%
Chromosomal syndrome defects	161,104	—	—	776	0.5%	160,328	99.5%
Other syndrome defects	161,104	—	—	776	0.5%	160,328	99.5%

[a]Births with a recorded gestation of less than 20 weeks or more than 50 weeks were excluded from the analysis.

We also tested the sensitivity of the results to numerous model specifications. The birth weight models were run with and without gestational age as a covariate, as well as with and without other potentially confounding variables. These variables were initially identified as potentially confounding in the sense that they might be related to the outcome and exposure with an unclear causal relationship. Model results for the reduced set of covariates (i.e., models without the confounding variables) for the prenatal development outcomes and infant mortality are presented in Appendix E. The birth defect models were similarly run with and without the "inadequate care" variable, the results of which are shown in Appendix F.

Because two potentially important covariates, mother's education and the number of previous infant deaths, were only available for the years 1989 to 1993, we ran models for this time period to test the effect of including these covariates on the exposure coefficients. Because including these two covariates had little effect on the exposure coefficients, the results are not presented in the report.

Power of Statistical Tests

For each outcome and exposure group, we estimated the minimum effect that the statistical tests could detect, given power of 80 percent.[14] The "minimum effect" is expressed as an odds ratio, defined as the ratio between the exposed and control groups of the odds of a particular adverse birth outcome occurring. The magnitude depends on the frequency of the outcome and sample size. For example, we determined that given the sample size and the base rate of 17 defects per 1,000 live births, we have power of 80 percent to detect an effect in the group with the lowest exposure, if the odds of any defect are 1.2 times higher for the exposed group than for the controls. The formula for the minimum odds ratio, OR_{min}, is given by

$$p_{exp} = \frac{3.92 + n_{exp}p_{cntl} + 2.8\sqrt{1.96 + n_{exp}p_{cntl}(1-p_{cntl}) + (7.84 + n_{exp})n_{exp}v_{cntl}}}{7.84 + n_{exp}}$$

$$v_{cntl} = \frac{p_{cntl}(1-p_{cntl})}{n_{cntl}}$$

$$OR_{min} = \frac{p_{exp}(1-p_{cntl})}{p_{cntl}(1-p_{exp})}$$

where p_{exp} is rate of adverse outcomes for the exposed group, n_{exp} is sample size for the exposed group and p_{cntl} and n_{cntl} are the corresponding values for the control group (Snedecor and Cochran, 1980).[15] For each of the outcomes in the study, we

---

[14]The power of a statistical test refers to the probability that the test will identify an effect (e.g., an odds ratio greater than 1) when it exists.

[15]The formula assumes that we are testing the difference in the raw rates. We are actually using logistic regression to conduct our test and adjusting for covariates. However, the power of our logistic regression–

calculated the minimum odds ratio that we have power of 80 percent to detect. We present the results of these power calculations in Appendix D and discuss them in Chapter Five.

---

based tests should be very similar to the power of a test for the difference in rates. We adjusted our power calculation to account for the possible correlation of births within a ZIP. For each outcome—prenatal development outcomes or defects—we estimated the standard error of our regression parameters of exposure both with and without an adjustment for possible correlations within a ZIP. The square of the ratio of these standard error estimates is an estimate of the loss of precision due to correlation within a ZIP, the design effect. For calculating power the design effect is equivalent to a loss of sample size, so we divided the true sample size by the design effect to determine the effective sample size that was used in our calculations.

Chapter Four

RESULTS

Rates of adverse birth outcomes were compared between two areas of Los Angeles County, one receiving reclaimed water and the other receiving no reclaimed water. The adverse birth outcomes include low birth weight, very low birth weight, preterm birth, infant mortality, all birth defects (excluding syndromes), all chromosomal syndromes, all syndromes other than chromosomal, and 16 specific types of birth defects. The pattern of results shows that rates of prenatal development outcomes and infant mortality between 1982 and 1993, infant mortality rates between 1982 and 1993, and rates of all types of birth defects between 1990 and 1993 were similar in the reclaimed water and control groups. The results in this report do not generally support the hypothesis of an association between residence in an area receiving reclaimed water and higher rates of these outcomes or with a dose-response relationship between reclaimed water and the rate of these outcomes.

CHARACTERISTICS OF STUDY POPULATIONS

Study Populations in 1990

A total of 1,006,487 people live in 22 Montebello Forebay ZIP codes receiving some percentage of reclaimed water in their water supplies during at least one year between 1982 and 1993. These ZIP codes represent more than 11 percent of the population of Los Angeles County (Table 4.1). According to the 1990 U.S. Census, more than 65 percent of the population receiving reclaimed water is Hispanic, with much smaller percentages of non-Hispanic whites, African-Americans, and Asians. Almost one-third of those living in the reclaimed water area are not U.S. citizens, more than in Los Angeles County as a whole. Compared to all of Los Angeles County, the reclaimed water area has a higher percentage of families living below the poverty level, a lower percentage of professional workers, and a much lower percentage of adults with a high school education or more. About half of residents of reclaimed water areas have lived in their residence for five years or more.

As described in Chapter Three, two locations were chosen to serve as a control area: the Pomona area and the northeastern San Fernando Valley. The 1990 population of the ZIP codes in the two control locations was 617,190, about 60 percent of the size of the population receiving reclaimed water. Together, the ZIP codes in the reclaimed water and control areas contain more than 18 percent of the population of Los Ange-

Table 4.1

Characteristics of Populations Living in the Reclaimed Water and Control Areas,
Based on the 1990 U.S. Census

Characteristic (in 1990)	Reclaimed Water Area[a]	Control Area	Los Angeles County
Population	1,006,487	617,190	8,863,164
Hispanic	65.5%	42.8%	37.3%
Non-Hispanic			
White	25.7%	41.5%	41.0%
Black	3.4%	6.9%	10.7%
Asian	4.8%	8.1%	10.4%
Persons 0–17 years	52.3%	43.3%	26.2%
Persons 65 years and older	14.7%	13.1%	9.7%
Persons who are not U.S. citizens	28.3%	27.6%	23.7%
Families below poverty level	12.7%	10.6%	11.6%
Employed in white-collar occupations	15.9%	22.8%	27.6%
Adults with eight years of education or less	25.4%	17.4%	15.6%
Adults with high school education or more	54.2%	66.7%	70.0%
Housing units that are renter-occupied	50.0%	47.8%	51.8%
Living in same house for at least five years	51.8%	42.9%	47.2%
Moved into current residence in 1989–1990	21.5%	25.9%	24.1%

[a]Several ZIP codes included in this column were not served any reclaimed water during one or
more years between 1982 and 1993. These can be identified using the data listed in Appendix B.

les County. Because the control area was matched to the reclaimed water area, most
demographic and socioeconomic characteristics are similar. Compared to the
reclaimed water area, however, the population in the control area is less Hispanic (43
percent versus 65 percent) with more non-Hispanic whites, African-Americans, and
Asians. Areas in Los Angeles County with a higher percentage of Hispanic persons
could not be used as a control group because of groundwater contamination (e.g.,
the San Gabriel Valley). In addition, the control area has a smaller proportion of
people who are not U.S. citizens, about the same percentage of families below
poverty level, and more white-collar workers and adults with a high school education
or more. About half of the residents of the control area had lived in the same house
for five years or longer.

CHARACTERISTICS OF BIRTHS IN STUDY POPULATIONS

As described in Chapter Three, for the purpose of analysis, each birth was assigned to
one of five groups based on the percentage of reclaimed water served to the ZIP code
of the mother's residence during the year of birth. These five groups are defined on
the basis of the percentage of reclaimed water: 0 percent, more than 0 to less than 2
percent, 2 to less than 5 percent, 5 to less than 15 percent, and 15 percent and higher.
These five groups are referred to as: control, RW 1, RW 2, RW 3, and RW 4, respectively, throughout the report.[1]

---

[1]The five categories are defined in Chapter Three. For all analyses, each birth was allocated to an exposure category based on the average annual percentage of reclaimed water in the year of birth.

All births occurring in a 12-year period (1982–1993) in the ZIP codes in the reclaimed water and control groups were included in the analyses of the prenatal development and infant mortality outcomes. The characteristics of the births in these analyses are shown in Table 4.2. Over the 12-year period, 452,275 births occurred in all study groups combined: 194,201 in the ZIP codes not receiving reclaimed water in the year of birth (i.e., the control group) and between 41,777 (RW 4) and 85,844 (RW 3) in the four reclaimed water groups. A high percentage of the infants in all these groups were born to Hispanic women, ranging from 62 percent of births in RW 2 to 88 percent of births in RW 1 classified as Hispanic. The characteristics of the births in RW 1 reflect the lower socioeconomic status of this population, with a higher percentage of young mothers and mothers receiving inadequate and/or late prenatal care. RW 4 also reflects the characteristics of a population with higher socioeconomic status— fewer births to young mothers and fewer women receiving care considered inadequate or late. Also, almost 60 percent of the mothers in RW 1 were born in Mexico, compared to about 40 percent in the control and other reclaimed water groups. The percentage of infants who are firstborn is also lowest in RW 1 and highest in RW 4.

Because birth defects–monitoring was initiated in mid-1990 in Los Angeles County, only those births occurring between July 1990 and December 1993 are included in the analyses of birth defects. The characteristics of the births in these analyses are shown in Table 4.3. Over the 3.5-year period, there were 160,328 births in these groups: 70,344 in the control group and between 21,167 (RW 1) to 26,405 (RW 4) in the reclaimed water groups. Many of the characteristics of the births occurring in the reclaimed water groups described in the paragraph above also apply to the births during this period. The level of the mothers' education in the RW 1 and RW 4 groups reflects their lower and higher socioeconomic status, respectively. [2]

ASSOCIATION BETWEEN RECLAIMED WATER AND OUTCOMES

The analysis of data in this report addresses the question of whether adverse birth outcomes are associated with residence in an area that receives reclaimed water. From the results, we are able to draw conclusions regarding how the rates in the reclaimed water group compare with rates in the control group: Are they higher, lower, or about the same? We are also able to report on how the rates vary in groups with increasing percentages of reclaimed water in their drinking water supplies. Even if the results indicate a strong association between reclaimed water and a specific adverse birth outcome, however, we cannot conclude that reclaimed water caused the outcome. Many other possible explanations for such results would have to be ruled out by conducting other types of studies. Conversely, if the results indicate no association between reclaimed water and a specific adverse birth outcome, we cannot conclude that reclaimed water causes no health effects among infants. Rather, we can only conclude that the effect is not large enough to be detected by this

---

[2]Mother's education was available for 1990–1993, but not available for the earlier years.

Table 4.2

Characteristics of Births Occurring Among Residents of Reclaimed Water and Control Areas, 1982–1993, by Percentage of Reclaimed Water

Percentage of Reclaimed Water	0% (Control)	Up to 2% (RW 1)	2–<5% (RW 2)	5–<15% (RW 3)	15% or more (RW 4)
Number of Births	194,201	73,088	57,365	85,844	41,777
			Percentage		
Race/Ethnicity of Mother					
Hispanic	62.3	88.1	62.1	73.8	75.5
Non-Hispanic					
White	25.9	8.3	24.5	18.8	18.4
Black	5.7	2.1	8.1	2.0	1.5
Asian	3.1	0.7	2.4	2.9	2.5
Other/unknown	3.0	0.9	2.9	2.6	2.1
Birthplace of Mother					
United States	42.2	33.2	47.3	43.0	50.0
Mexico	38.4	59.4	40.9	42.5	37.1
Other/unknown	19.6	7.4	11.8	14.5	12.9
Age of Mother					
Less than 20	12.2	15.2	14.0	13.7	13.1
20–34	78.8	76.3	78.8	78.6	77.9
35 and older	9.0	8.5	7.2	7.7	9.0
Male Child	51.2	51.1	51.5	51.4	50.8
First-Born	39.9	36.6	37.7	38.5	40.4
Previous Infant Death(s)					
None	97.8	97.5	97.9	98.0	98.2
One or more	2.2	2.5	2.1	2.0	1.7
Missing	0.1	0.1	0.1	0.1	0.1
Interval Since Last Birth					
Less than one year	2.0	2.4	2.2	2.1	2.0
One year or more	57.7	60.4	59.5	58.8	57.3
First-born/missing	40.3	37.2	38.3	39.1	40.7
Trimester Prenatal Care Begun After					
First	71.1	67.4	69.9	69.4	75.2
Second	23.3	26.0	23.7	24.5	20.4
Third trimester or never	5.6	6.7	6.4	6.1	4.4
Cardiac or Kidney Disease in Mother					
Yes	0.4	0.3	0.3	0.3	0.4
Unknown	99.6	99.7	99.7	99.7	99.6

type of study, or the effect was not detected for other reasons, such as exposure misclassification or inability to control for some differences among the groups.

PATTERNS OF HEALTH OUTCOMES IN STUDY POPULATIONS

Hypotheses Tested

Using a cohort study design, we tested the hypotheses that rates of adverse birth outcomes are the same in areas with reclaimed water and similar areas receiving no

Table 4.3

Characteristics of Births Occurring Among Residents of Reclaimed Water and Control Areas, July 1990–December 1993, by Percentage of Reclaimed Water

Percentage of Reclaimed Water	0% (Control)	Up to 2% (RW 1)	2–<5% (RW 2)	5–<15% (RW 3)	15% or more (RW 4)
Number of Births	70,334	21,167	18,502	23,920	26,405
			Percentage		
Race/Ethnicity of Mother					
Hispanic	72.1	92.3	70.8	80.5	82.0
Non-Hispanic					
White	17.5	6.0	15.5	12.1	12.5
Black	4.7	0.6	9.1	2.7	1.6
Asian	2.7	0.6	1.9	2.2	2.3
Other/missing	2.9	0.6	2.6	2.6	1.7
Age of Mother					
Less than 20	12.7	15.2	14.6	14.9	13.5
20–34	77.1	75.6	77.1	76.6	76.9
35 and older	10.2	9.2	8.3	8.5	9.6
Male Child	51.2	50.8	51.4	51.2	50.4
Education of Mother					
Less than high school	26.9	33.1	25.2	24.7	18.3
High school	50.1	54.1	56.6	58.6	59.4
College or higher	23.0	12.8	18.2	16.7	22.4
Quality of Prenatal Care					
Inadequate	8.4	10.8	9.8	10.1	7.6
Unknown	91.7	89.2	90.2	89.9	92.4

reclaimed water. The analyses are aimed specifically at comparing rates of low birth weight, preterm birth, infant mortality, and birth defects using existing data. For each adverse birth outcome, we compared births in each of the four reclaimed water groups with births in the control group.

Measures of Exposure Effect and Statistical Significance

For each health outcome, an odds ratio and a confidence interval around the odds ratio were calculated using the parameter estimates generated by the logistic regression model. The odds ratio is a measure of association commonly used in epidemiology. In this study, an odds ratio of greater than 1.0 indicates the rate is higher in the reclaimed water group than in the control group. An odds ratio less of than 1.0 indicates the rate is lower in the reclaimed water group than in the control group. The estimated odds ratios are used to evaluate whether the rates in the four groups with reclaimed water differ from the rate in the control group.

The upper and lower bounds of the 95 percent confidence interval (CI) represent a range of possible values for the odds ratio given the uncertainties associated with the data.[3] A direct relationship exists between the confidence interval and statistical significance. If the 95 percent confidence interval does not include the value of 1.0, the difference between the reclaimed water and control groups could be labeled as "statistically significant" (using the traditional p-value of 0.05). The confidence interval also provides information on the uncertainty associated with the estimate as well as the size of the effect—the wider the confidence interval, the more uncertain the estimate.

The results from every statistical comparison performed in the study are presented in this report. An alternative approach would be to present only those results that are statistically significant. Presenting the results of all statistical tests is highly recommended by Thomas et al. (1985). In these comparisons, a fixed alpha level[4] of 0.05 has been assumed for all statistical tests.

Statistical significance is a tool that allows us to judge how probable or improbable a particular result is, but it reveals nothing about cause and effect. Using statistical significance as the only criterion to decide whether a result is important may focus attention on the wrong subset of results. Some small (and perhaps meaningless) differences may be statistically significant because they are based on large sample sizes, whereas some large (and perhaps meaningful) differences may not be statistically significant because they are based on small sample sizes. Because statistical significance is highly dependent on sample size, other criteria should also be considered in evaluating whether an association between an exposure and a health outcome is important or causal. Statistical significance is often used in epidemiology and other disciplines that use hypothesis-testing to highlight the "most important" results. Although statistical significance should not be the only criterion used in judging which results are most important, its widespread acceptance as a standard of importance justifies some discussion of its occurrence and meaning in the context of this study.

Assessing Causality of Associations

If an association between reclaimed water and a health outcome is found in an epidemiologic study, it is important to consider whether the association is spurious or may indicate a causal relationship.[5] In attempting to distinguish between causal and noncausal associations, several aspects of the association should be considered. Among these are strength, consistency, temporality, biologic gradient, plausibility, and coherence (Rothman, 1986; Hill, 1965).

The "strength" of an association refers to the magnitude of the odds ratio. In this study, odds ratios greater than 2.0 would be considered more indicative of a causal

---

[3]A "95 percent confidence interval around the odds ratio" can be interpreted as follows: If a study based on this type of data was repeated in a similar population, the confidence intervals based on 95 percent of the replications would include the "true value" of the odds ratio, given the variability in the data.

[4]The alpha level or Type I error is the probability of finding a difference when in fact there is no difference. The level of acceptance of Type I error in a test of statistical significance is called the alpha.

[5]This discussion is taken from the report on the Phase 1 study (Sloss et al., 1996).

association between reclaimed water and a health outcome than odds ratios between 1.0 and 2.0, although the latter may also be of interest. "Consistency" of an association refers to the recurrence of the same finding under different circumstances (e.g., in studies of different populations at different times). If a relationship between reclaimed water and a health outcome were causal, results from studies conducted in different geographic areas or during different periods of time would be expected to yield the same result. The issue of consistency must be evaluated between the results of this study and two other sets of results: previous studies of the same population and studies of other populations that tested related hypotheses.

"Temporality" of an association means that the cause must come before the effect. In this study, any adverse birth outcome occurring during the study period (1982–1993) comes after the introduction of groundwater recharge with reclaimed water in 1962 in the Montebello Forebay and therefore would satisfy the criterion of temporality. The "biologic gradient" refers to a relationship between the cause and effect that follows a dose response curve, with a larger effect (or response) occurring as a result of a larger exposure (or dose). If reclaimed water causes a particular type of health effect, rates would be expected to be higher in a group with more reclaimed water than in a group with less reclaimed water.

"Plausibility" of the association refers to the biological basis for an association between a particular cause and an effect. In the case of reclaimed water, plausibility is difficult to demonstrate because no cause (e.g., a "potentially harmful" substance in reclaimed water) has been identified. If an increased rate of lung cancer were to be found in the reclaimed water groups, it would be highly implausible that reclaimed water caused the lung cancer to occur, given what is known about the causes and biology of lung cancer. It is plausible, however, that exposure to an environmental contaminant might result in an adverse birth outcome.

"Coherence" of an association refers to how well the scientific evidence supports an association between a cause and effect. This is similar to the plausibility criterion but refers to the fact that interpreting an association as a cause-and-effect phenomenon should not conflict with accepted facts about the natural history and biology of the disease (Rothman, 1986). Each of these criteria is important in evaluating the causal nature of an association.

The dose-response criterion is of particular interest when studying the health effects of reclaimed water. The wide range of exposure to reclaimed water in the populations being studied (from a minimum of 0 to a maximum of 38 percent reclaimed water in the water supplies) allows evaluation of a dose-response effect. If reclaimed water were causing a health effect, a dose-response relationship might be expected, with higher odds ratios in groups having higher percentages of reclaimed water.[6]

---

[6]An alternative model might assume a "threshold effect" with a threshold value above which a constant effect (i.e., of the same magnitude) is observed.

PRENATAL DEVELOPMENT AND INFANT MORTALITY

Adjusted odds ratios and confidence intervals were calculated for four measures of prenatal development: low birth weight (infants weighing less than 2,500 grams at birth) among full-term births (37–41 weeks of gestation), low birth weight among all births (20–50 weeks of gestation), very low birth weight (infants weighing less than 1,500 grams at birth) among all births, and preterm birth (births occurring at less than 37 weeks of gestation) (Table 4.4). The unadjusted (or crude) rates for each group are also shown in Table 4.4. These measures are based on information derived from birth certificates for the 12-year period from 1982–1993. As described above, every birth was classified into one of four reclaimed water groups or the control group based on the annual percentage of reclaimed water received by the ZIP code of the mother's residence at the time of birth. The number of cases of each outcome

Table 4.4

Adjusted Odds Ratios for Prenatal Development Outcomes and Infant Mortality by Percentage of Reclaimed Water, Los Angeles County, 1982–1993

Outcome and Percentage of Reclaimed Water	Number of Cases	Unadjusted Rate (per 1,000 births)	Adjusted Odds Ratio[a]	95% Confidence Interval
Low Birth Weight (full-term only)				
0% (Control)	3,765	26.42	1.00	NA
More than 0 to <2% (RW 1)	1,316	24.78	0.98	0.90–1.06
2–<5% (RW 2)	1,086	26.20	0.95	0.89–1.01
5–<15% (RW 3)	1,517	24.39	0.96	0.90–1.02
15% or higher (RW 4)	691	22.15	0.88[b]	0.81–0.96
Low Birth Weight (all births)				
0% (Control)	9,003	46.88	1.00	NA
More than 0 to <2% (RW 1)	3,181	44.11	0.97	0.91–1.04
2–<5% (RW 2)	2,644	46.71	0.92[b]	0.88–0.96
5–<15% (RW 3)	3,635	42.88	0.93[b]	0.88–0.98
15% or higher (RW 4)	1,753	42.25	0.91[b]	0.84–0.98
Very Low Birth Weight				
0% (Control)	1,457	7.59	1.00	NA
More than 0 to <2% (RW 1)	503	6.97	0.85[b]	0.75–0.96
2–<5% (RW 2)	442	7.81	0.90	0.76–1.07
5–<15% (RW 3)	639	7.54	1.07	0.92–1.24
15% or higher (RW 4)	308	7.42	1.00	0.89–1.13
Preterm Birth				
0% (Control)	14,810	77.08	1.00	NA
More than 0 to <2% (RW 1)	5,626	77.96	0.98	0.93–1.04
2–<5% (RW 2)	4,635	81.85	1.03	0.95–1.11
5–<15% (RW 3)	6,639	78.28	1.02	0.97–1.06
15% or higher (RW 4)	3,121	75.20	0.99	0.94–1.05
Infant Mortality				
0% (Control)	1,335	6.75	1.00	NA
More than 0 to <2% (RW 1)	521	7.00	1.05	0.92–1.21
2–<5% (RW 2)	438	7.49	1.05	0.92–1.19
5–<15% (RW 3)	597	6.81	1.04	0.90–1.19
15% or higher (RW 4)	225	5.28	0.82[b]	0.73–0.92

[a]Based on logistic regression adjusted for maternal race/ethnicity, maternal age, gender of child, median housing value, birthplace of mother, birth order, maternal medical problems (cardiac, kidney), weeks of gestation, birth interval, month prenatal care began, and previous infant deaths.
[b]Statistically significant (p<0.05).

can be found in Table 4.4 along with the odds ratios and confidence intervals comparing the rates in the four reclaimed water groups with the rate in the control group. These analyses control statistically for maternal race/ethnicity, maternal age, gender of child, median housing value by ZIP code, birthplace of mother, birth order of child, maternal medical problems, length of gestation, birth interval, month prenatal care began, and number of previous infant deaths. The odds ratios for all variables in this model (labeled as Model 1) are shown in Appendix E. In addition, Appendix E contains results for three other models:

- Model 2: Same set of covariates as Model 1; control group defined as San Fernando Valley only.

- Model 3: Demographic covariates only; control group defined as San Fernando Valley and Pomona.

- Model 4: Demographic covariates only; control group defined as San Fernando Valley only.

The odds ratios for low birth weight (LBW) are slightly less than 1.0 (0.88 to 0.98) for the four reclaimed water groups, indicating that the rates of low birth weight are slightly lower than in the control group (Table 4.4). The pattern of results for LBW is similar when the analysis is restricted to full-term births, with odds ratios ranging from 0.91 to 0.97. There is no indication that the odds ratios for LBW increase with increasing percentages of reclaimed water for either subset of births. The odds ratios for very low birth weight (VLBW) range in magnitude from 0.85 (RW 1) to 1.07 (RW 3), indicating no association between this outcome and the percentage of reclaimed water. There is also no increasing trend in VLBW odds ratios with increasing percentages of reclaimed water. The odds ratios for preterm birth are close to 1.0, ranging from 0.98 (RW 1) to 1.03 (RW 2), indicating that rates of infants born prematurely in the four reclaimed water groups are similar to each other and the control group (Table 4.4). There is no evidence of an increasing trend in preterm birth with increasing reclaimed water.

Odds ratios and confidence intervals were calculated for deaths during the first year of life among infants in the reclaimed water and control groups. Deaths due to accidents and injuries (ICD-9 codes 800–999) were considered unrelated to reclaimed water or any other environmental exposure and, therefore, were not included in these analyses. The odds ratios in the four reclaimed water groups ranged from 0.82 (RW 4) to 1.05 (RW 1 and RW 2). Based on these results, the odds ratios for infant mortality do not appear to be increasing with increasing percentages of reclaimed water.

BIRTH DEFECTS

The results of the analyses of birth defects data for a 3.5-year period (July 1990–December 1993) are shown in Tables 4.5 through 4.9. We present the adjusted odds ratios and confidence intervals based on the multiple logistic regression models for an infant having any type of defect and for an infant having a particular type of defect. The unadjusted (or crude) rates for each group are also shown in Tables 4.5

through 4.9.   These analyses control statistically for year of birth, maternal race/ethnicity, maternal age, gender of child, education of mother, and adequacy of prenatal care. Odds ratios for all variables in this model are shown in Appendix F, labeled as Model 1. In addition, Appendix F contains results for three other models:

- Model 2: Same set of covariates as Model 1; control group defined as San Fernando Valley only.

- Model 3: Demographic covariates only; control group defined as San Fernando Valley and Pomona.

- Model 4: Demographic covariates only; control group defined as San Fernando Valley only.

In reviewing these results, the reader should keep in mind that birth defects among liveborn infants represent a subset of all birth defects, many of which result in adverse outcomes before birth.[7] We must assume that the proportion of infants with a birth defect who survive the gestational period and are born alive does not differ between the reclaimed water and control groups. If this assumption is accepted, comparing the rate of birth defects among liveborn infants seems to be a reasonable proxy for the rate of birth defects among all pregnancies.

All Birth Defects, Neural Tube, Other Nervous System, and Eyes, Ears, Face, and Neck Defects

In the analysis of all birth defects, infants with any single birth defect (as well as more than one defect) were classified as having the outcome.[8] Although odds ratios for RW 1, RW 3, and RW 4 are slightly below 1.0 and RW 2 is slightly above 1.0, all of the odds ratios for all defects are close to 1.0 (Table 4.5). This pattern indicates that the risk of having a birth defect diagnosed during the first year of life, regardless of type, is similar between the reclaimed water groups and the control group, with no evidence of an increasing dose-response relationship.[9]

For neural tube defects,[10] the odds ratios range from 1.44 to 1.52 for the three reclaimed water groups with less than 15 percent reclaimed water (RW 1, RW 2, and RW 3), meaning they are elevated compared to the control group. The odds ratio for RW 4 is less than 1.0, indicating that the rate is lower than for the other three reclaimed water groups and less than the control group. The odds ratio for RW 4, however, is based on 8 cases, and, therefore, cannot be considered reliable. The

---

[7]The CBDMP collects available information on birth defects identified among stillborn infants. Because information on all pregnancies is not available, however, we chose to limit the analyses to birth defects identified in liveborn infants.

[8] This analysis excluded infants classified as having defects constituting a "syndrome."

[9]An environmental toxin is unlikely to cause an increase in all defects.

[10] The category of neural tube defects includes spina bifida and anencephalus.

Table 4.5

Adjusted Odds Ratios for All Birth Defects, Nervous System Defects, and Defects of Ears, Eyes, Face, and Neck by Percentage of Reclaimed Water, Los Angeles County, 1990–1993

Outcome and Percentage of Reclaimed Water	Number of Cases	Unadjusted Rate (per 1,000 births)	Adjusted Odds Ratio[a]	95% Confidence Interval
All Defects				
0% (Control)	1,165	16.61	1.00	NA
More than 0 to <2% (RW 1)	331	15.68	0.98	0.87–1.11
2–<5% (RW 2)	317	17.19	1.04	0.87–1.23
5–<15% (RW 3)	368	15.43	0.94	0.83–1.06
15% or higher (RW 4)	390	14.82	0.92	0.81–1.03
Neural Tube Defects				
0% (Control)	27	0.39	1.00	NA
More than 0 to <2% (RW 1)	14	0.66	1.52[b]	1.03–2.24
2–<5% (RW 2)	10	0.54	1.44	0.90–2.29
5–<15% (RW 3)	15	0.63	1.55	0.96–2.50
15% or higher (RW 4)	8	0.30	0.81	0.21–3.04
Other Nervous System Defects				
0% (Control)	133	1.90	1.00	NA
More than 0 to <2% (RW 1)	46	2.18	1.19	0.84–1.69
2–<5% (RW 2)	37	2.01	1.04	0.77–1.42
5–<15% (RW 3)	49	2.05	1.10	0.77–1.58
15% or higher (RW 4)	41	1.56	0.89	0.66–1.19
Ears, Eyes, Face, Neck Defects				
0% (Control)	260	3.71	1.00	NA
More than 0 to <2% (RW 1)	70	3.32	0.86	0.69–1.06
2–<5% (RW 2)	91	4.93	1.34[b]	1.08–1.66
5–<15% (RW 3)	80	3.35	0.88	0.70–1.10
15% or higher (RW 4)	87	3.30	0.89	0.73–1.09

[a]Based on logistic regression adjusted for year of birth, maternal race/ethnicity, maternal age, gender of child, education of mother, and adequacy of prenatal care.

[b]Statistically significant (p<0.05).

pattern for other defects of the nervous system[11] is similar to that for neural tube defects, but the odds ratios are closer to 1.0. The odds ratios for RW 1, RW 2, and RW 3 range from 1.04 to 1.19, and the lowest odds ratio (0.89) is for RW 4. The pattern does not conform to a traditional dose-response relationship.[12] The odds ratio for defects of the ears, eyes, face, and neck for RW 2 is 1.34. Odds ratios range from 0.86 to 0.89 for the other three reclaimed water groups. The overall pattern of results for ears, eyes, face, and neck defects does not support the hypothesis of a dose-response relationship.

---

[11]Nervous system defects included in this category are encephalocele, microcephalus, reduction deformities of the brain, hydrocephalus, and other anomalies of the brain and spinal cord.

[12]Neural tube defects and defects of the nervous system can be detected through the use of prenatal amniocentesis testing. If the rate of amniocentesis differed between births in the reclaimed water categories and the control category, the rate of elective abortion might also differ, thus lowering the rates of these defects in categories with higher rates of amniocentesis. This could not be evaluated in this study.

Table 4.6

Adjusted Odds Ratios for Cardiac Defects and Respiratory System Defects by
Percentage of Reclaimed Water, Los Angeles County, 1990–1993

Outcome and Percentage of Reclaimed Water	Number of Cases	Unadjusted Rate (per 1,000 births)	Adjusted Odds Ratio[a]	95% Confidence Interval
Major Cardiac Defects				
0% (Control)	196	2.80	1.00	NA
More than 0 to <2% (RW 1)	65	3.08	1.17[b]	1.01–1.35
2–<5% (RW 2)	47	2.55	0.92	0.72–1.17
5–<15% (RW 3)	74	3.10	1.14	0.92–1.42
15% or higher (RW 4)	84	3.19	1.23	0.94–1.61
Patent Ductus Arteriosus				
0% (Control)	66	0.94	1.00	NA
More than 0 to <2% (RW 1)	23	1.09	1.34	0.94–1.90
2–<5% (RW 2)	17	0.92	1.03	0.72–1.48
5–<15% (RW 3)	25	1.05	1.14	0.77–1.70
15% or higher (RW 4)	28	1.06	1.28	0.84–1.97
Other Cardiac Defects				
0% (Control)	106	1.51	1.00	NA
More than 0 to <2% (RW 1)	31	1.47	0.98	0.65–1.49
2–<5% (RW 2)	24	1.03	0.85	0.58–1.25
5–<15% (RW 3)	38	1.59	1.05	0.73–1.51
15% or higher (RW 4)	31	1.18	0.80	0.56–1.15
Respiratory System Defects				
0% (Control)	125	1.78	1.00	NA
More than 0 to <2% (RW 1)	39	1.85	1.05	0.78–1.42
2–<5% (RW 2)	41	2.22	1.24	0.91–1.70
5–<15% (RW 3)	48	2.01	1.11	0.85–1.45
15% or higher (RW 4)	48	1.82	1.04	0.76–1.44

[a]Based on logistic regression adjusted for year of birth, maternal race/ethnicity, maternal age, gender of child, education of mother, and adequacy of prenatal care.

[b]Statistically significant (p<0.05).

Major Cardiac Defects, Patent Ductus Arteriosus, Other Cardiac, and Respiratory System Defects

The odds ratios for major cardiac defects are 1.14, 1.17, and 1.23 for RW 3, RW 1, and RW 4, respectively, and 0.92 for RW 2 (Table 4.6). The pattern of results does not conform to a dose-response relation, but might indicate a slight overall increase for the reclaimed water groups. The odds ratios for the cardiac defect, patent ductus arteriosus,[13] are higher than 1.0 for all four reclaimed water groups, ranging from 1.03 (RW 2) to 1.34 (RW 1). The pattern of odds ratios is not consistent with a dose-response relationship.

For other cardiac defects, RW 1, RW 2, and RW 4 have odds ratios of less than 1.0 (0.98, 0.85, and 0.80, respectively) and RW 3 has an odds ratio of slightly higher than 1.0 (1.05). For defects of the respiratory system, the odds ratios for all four of the reclaimed water groups are slightly higher than 1.0, ranging from 1.04 (RW 4) to 1.24

---

[13]This defect was analyzed separately from the other cardiac defects because it occurs commonly among premature infants and, therefore, is considered an outcome secondary to preterm birth.

(RW 2). For other cardiac and respiratory system defects, the magnitudes of the odds ratios indicate the rates are similar between the reclaimed water and control groups and show a pattern inconsistent with an increasing dose-response relationship.

Cleft Defects, Pyloric Stenosis, Intestinal Atresias, and Other Digestive System Defects

RW 1, RW 3, and RW 4 have odds ratios for the cleft defects[14] that are higher than 1.0 (1.13, 1.09, and 1.10, respectively) (Table 4.7). The odds ratio for RW 2 is 0.82. There is not a pattern of increasing magnitude that would provide evidence of an association with reclaimed water.

The results for three digestive system defects are also shown in Table 4.7. For pyloric stenosis,[15] the odds ratios for RW 1 and RW 4 are higher than 1.0 (1.03 and 1.09, respectively) and odds ratios for RW 2 and RW 3 are less than 1.0 (0.94 and 0.77, respectively). The odds ratios for intestinal atresias[16] are 1.04 and 1.15 for RW 1 and RW 3 (respectively), and 0.85 and 0.71 for RW 2 and RW 4. The odds ratios for other digestive system defects are higher than 1.0 for the four reclaimed water groups, ranging from 1.07 (RW 4) to 1.40 (RW 2). This indicates a slight increase in risk for all of the reclaimed water groups. The magnitudes and patterns of the odds ratios for the first two digestive defect categories are not consistent with the hypothesis of a dose-response effect. However, the other digestive defects appear to be consistently elevated in the reclaimed water groups.

For defects of the urogenital system (Table 4.7), RW 1 and RW 2 have odds ratios slightly above 1.0 (1.18 and 1.03, respectively) whereas RW 3 and RW 4 have odds ratios slightly below 1.0 (0.91 and 0.98, respectively). These odds ratios for defects of the urogenital system do not suggest an association with reclaimed water.

Limb, Other Musculoskeletal, Integument, and All Other Defects

The odds ratios for limb defects[17] are close to or above 1.0 for all four reclaimed water groups, ranging from 0.99 (RW 2) to 2.08 (RW 3) (Table 4.8). The higher odds ratios in RW 3 and RW 4 indicate an increasing trend with reclaimed water and are consistent with a dose-response or threshold effect. For all four groups, these results are based on small numbers of cases (between 7 and 14 defects).

The odds ratios for "other musculoskeletal defects"[18] are slightly less than 1.0 for RW 1 (0.84) and RW 4 (0.93) and slightly above 1.0 for RW 2 (1.16) and RW 3 (1.01)

---

[14]The category of cleft defects includes cleft palate and cleft lip.

[15]Pyloric stenosis is an obstruction of the stomach.

[16]Intestinal atresias are obstructions of the upper or lower intestine.

[17]The category of limb defects includes absence and shortening of upper and lower limbs.

[18]The category of other musculoskeletal defects includes deformities of the skull, face, jaw, and feet; clubfoot; extra fingers or toes; webbed fingers or toes; and many other musculoskeletal defects.

Table 4.7

Adjusted Odds Ratios for Oral Cleft Defects, Digestive System Defects, and Urogenital System Defects by Percentage of Reclaimed Water, Los Angeles County, 1990–1993

Outcome and Percentage of Reclaimed Water	Number of Cases	Unadjusted Rate (per 1,000 births)	Adjusted Odds Ratio[a]	95% Confidence Interval
Cleft Defects				
0% (Control)	75	1.07	1.00	NA
More than 0 to <2% (RW 1)	26	1.23	1.13	0.62–2.07
2–<5% (RW 2)	16	0.87	0.82	0.57–1.17
5–<15% (RW 3)	28	1.17	1.09	0.79–1.51
15% or higher (RW 4)	31	1.18	1.10	0.80–1.50
Pyloric Stenosis				
0% (Control)	97	1.38	1.00	NA
More than 0 to <2% (RW 1)	30	1.42	1.03	0.78–1.35
2–<5% (RW 2)	24	1.30	0.94	0.71–1.26
5–<15% (RW 3)	26	1.09	0.77	0.53–1.13
15% or higher (RW 4)	41	1.56	1.09	0.82–1.45
Intestinal Atresias				
0% (Control)	49	0.70	1.00	NA
More than 0 to <2% (RW 1)	15	0.71	1.04	0.62–1.74
2–<5% (RW 2)	11	0.60	0.85	0.54–1.34
5–<15% (RW 3)	18	0.75	1.15	0.83–1.58
15% or higher (RW 4)	12	0.46	0.71	0.42–1.21
Other Digestive Systems Defects				
0% (Control)	152	2.17	1.00	NA
More than 0 to <2% (RW 1)	54	2.56	1.20	0.86–1.68
2–<5% (RW 2)	56	3.04	1.40[b]	1.15–1.72
5–<15% (RW 3)	58	2.43	1.11	0.91–1.37
15% or higher (RW 4)	60	2.28	1.07	0.75–1.53
Urogenital System Defects				
0% (Control)	237	3.38	1.00	NA
More than 0 to <2% (RW 1)	74	3.51	1.18	0.97–1.45
2–<5% (RW 2)	64	3.47	1.03	0.70–1.52
5–<15% (RW 3)	69	2.89	0.91	0.72–1.14
15% or higher (RW 4)	82	3.12	0.98	0.73–1.31

[a]Based on logistic regression adjusted for year of birth, maternal race/ethnicity, maternal age, gender of child, education of mother, and adequacy of prenatal care.

[b]Statistically significant ($p < 0.05$).

(Table 4.8). For defects of the integument,[19] the odds ratios for RW 1, RW 3, and RW 4 are lower than 1.0, ranging from 0.69 to 0.74, whereas the odds ratio for RW 2 is 1.13. Neither of these patterns of odds ratios support the hypothesis of an association with reclaimed water.

For the category of all other defects,[20] the odds ratios are above 1.0 for RW 1 and RW 3 (2.05 and 1.56, respectively) and below 1.0 for RW 2 and RW 4 (0.66 and 0.84) (Table 4.8). Although it appears that the rates in RW 1 and RW 3 are higher than in the

---

[19]This category includes anomalies of the hair, skin, and nails.

[20]This category includes anomalies of the spleen, adrenal gland, pituitary gland, and thyroid and parathyroid glands and other defects.

control group, these odds ratios do not follow a pattern consistent with an increasing dose-response relationship.

Chromosomal Syndromes and Syndromes Other Than Chromosomal

Syndromes are multiple defects that occur together in an individual infant and have been identified and recognized as a specific medical condition that has occurred repeatedly. Infants with defects classified as syndromes are analyzed separately because these defects may differ in etiology from defects that do not occur as syndromes.

The odds ratios for chromosomal syndromes are above 1.0 for RW 2, RW 3, and RW 4, ranging from 1.09 to 1.13 (Table 4.9). RW 1 has an odds ratio of 0.69. The pattern of results for chromosomal indicates somewhat higher risk in RW 3 and RW 4.

For syndromes other than chromosomal, RW 2 and RW 4 have odds ratios below 1.0 (0.88 and 0.89, respectively) and RW 1 and RW 3 have odds ratios above 1.0 (1.17 and

Table 4.8

Adjusted Odds Ratios for Musculoskeletal System Defects, Integument Defects, and All Other Defects by Percentage of Reclaimed Water, Los Angeles County, 1990–1993

Outcome and Percentage of Reclaimed Water	Number of Cases	Unadjusted Rate (per 1,000 births)	Adjusted Odds Ratio[a]	95% Confidence Interval
Limb Defects				
0% (Control)	19	0.27	1.00	NA
More than 0 to <2% (RW 1)	7	0.33	1.02	0.47–2.22
2–<5% (RW 2)	5	0.27	0.99	0.45–2.15
5–<15% (RW 3)	14	0.59	2.08[b]	1.48–2.91
15% or higher (RW 4)	10	0.38	1.38	0.79–2.44
Other Musculoskeletal Defects				
0% (Control)	405	5.78	1.00	NA
More than 0 to <2% (RW 1)	99	4.69	0.84	0.66–1.06
2–<5% (RW 2)	123	6.67	1.16	0.93–1.44
5–<15% (RW 3)	138	5.79	1.01	0.81–1.26
15% or higher (RW 4)	137	5.20	0.93	0.72–1.20
Integument Defects				
0% (Control)	214	3.05	1.00	NA
More than 0 to <2% (RW 1)	45	2.13	0.69[b]	0.49–0.99
2–<5% (RW 2)	63	3.42	1.13	0.74–1.75
5–<15% (RW 3)	55	2.31	0.74	0.52–1.05
15% or higher (RW 4)	56	2.13	0.71	0.48–1.06
All Other Defects				
0% (Control)	22	0.31	1.00	NA
More than 0 to <2% (RW 1)	15	0.71	2.05[b]	1.09–3.83
2–<5% (RW 2)	4	0.22	0.66	0.24–1.80
5–<15% (RW 3)	12	0.50	1.56	0.71–3.44
15% or higher (RW 4)	7	0.27	0.84	0.37–1.92

[a]Based on logistic regression adjusted for year of birth, maternal race/ethnicity, maternal age, gender of child, education of mother, and adequacy of prenatal care.
[b]Statistically significant ($p<0.05$).

1.01, respectively) (Table 4.9). The odds ratios do not conform to a pattern consistent with an increasing dose-response relationship.

Sensitivity Analyses

Sensitivity analyses were conducted to assess the effect of alternative conditions on the results.[21] The results presented in tables throughout this chapter are based on models that control for the characteristics most likely to affect the outcome rates. In addition, these models are based on a control area located in two locations, the San Fernando Valley and Pomona. Three alternative models were tested to assess the sensitivity of the results to including fewer variables in the regression model and using a different control area. The three alternative models are Model 2, using only the San Fernando Valley as the control area, with the same set of variables as in Model 1; Model 3, the same control area, but controlling only for demographic characteristics; and Model 4, using only the San Fernando Valley as the control area and controlling only for demographic characteristics. The model parameters for all four types of models are shown in Appendix E for the prenatal development outcomes and infant mortality and in Appendix F for birth defects.

To assess the sensitivity of the results to the covariates included in the model and the choice of control locations, we compared the results from these three alternative models with the results presented in this chapter. In general, the differences in results among the four models are minor and will not affect the conclusions of the

Table 4.9

Adjusted Odds Ratios for Chromosomal Defect Syndromes and All Other Defect Syndromes by Percentage of Reclaimed Water, Los Angeles County, 1990–1993

Outcome and Percentage of Reclaimed Water	Number of Cases	Unadjusted Rate (per 1,000 births)	Adjusted Odds Ratio[a]	95% Confidence Interval
Chromosomal Syndromes				
0% (Control)	142	2.02	1.00	NA
More than 0 to <2% (RW 1)	30	1.42	0.69[b]	0.48–0.98
2–<5% (RW 2)	39	2.11	1.10	0.78–1.55
5–<15% (RW 3)	50	2.09	1.09	0.86–1.37
15% or higher (RW 4)	58	2.20	1.13	0.81–1.58
Syndromes Other Than Chromosomal				
0% (Control)	71	1.01	1.00	NA
More than 0 to <2% (RW 1)	27	1.28	1.17	0.69–1.99
2–<5% (RW 2)	17	0.92	0.88	0.64–1.20
5–<15% (RW 3)	25	1.05	1.01	0.68–1.50
15% or higher (RW 4)	24	0.91	0.89	0.53–1.48

[a]Based on logistic regression adjusted for year of birth, maternal race/ethnicity, maternal age, gender of child, education of mother, and adequacy of prenatal care.
[b]Statistically significant ($p<0.05$).

---

[21]The rationale behind the sensitivity analyses is discussed in Chapter Three.

report. The overall pattern of results and the magnitude of the odds ratios remain generally unchanged by the alternative models, indicating that the patterns observed in the set of models presented in this chapter are not changed by controlling for fewer variables in the models (Models 3 and 4) or by using an alternative control area (Models 2 and 4). Most of the statistically significant results presented in this chapter remain statistically significant under the three alternative models. For the numerical results from Models 2 through 4, see Appendixes E and F.

In addition to these four models, we tested models for the 17 birth defects that collapsed the four "exposed" groups (i.e., RW 1–RW 4) into a single "exposed" group. We found no significant differences between the single exposed group and the control group when the models were run in this manner.

Chapter Five

SUMMARY AND DISCUSSION

The epidemiologic study reported here measures the association between adverse birth outcomes from 1982 to 1993 and residence in an area being served reclaimed water in Los Angeles County. The outcomes include four related to prenatal development (low birth weight among full-term births, low birth weight among all births, very low birth weight among all births, and preterm birth), infant mortality for the 12-year period from 1982 to 1993, and 19 categories of birth defects for a 3.5-year period from 1990 to 1993.

SUMMARY OF RESULTS

In general, the pattern of results does not provide evidence that supports an association between residence in an area receiving reclaimed water and prenatal development outcomes, infant mortality, or birth defects. Compared with the control group, the reclaimed water groups had somewhat higher rates for some of these adverse birth outcomes and somewhat lower rates for others. If reclaimed water led to an increase in any of these outcomes, the results would be expected to show some evidence of a dose-response relationship in which the outcome rates increase with increasingly more reclaimed water. The results in this report follow no such pattern. The limitations of the study, however, must be kept in mind when interpreting these results. These include the possibility of a biological model other than dose-response (e.g., a threshold model), exposure misclassification, and the limited ability of the study to detect an effect (i.e., power).

Prenatal Development. Overall, the adverse prenatal development outcomes occurred at about the same rate or less frequently in the reclaimed water groups than in the control group. RW 1 does not have higher risks than the control group generally and was very similar to RW 2 and RW 3. Several of the odds ratios for the prenatal development outcomes were statistically significantly lower than 1.0. RW 4, the group with the highest percentage of reclaimed water, had significantly lower odds ratios for low birth weight (among full-term births and all births) and for infant mortality.[1] This finding could be attributable to the inability of the study to control completely for many differences (e.g., personal health habits) among the areas.

---

[1] The lower odds ratios for these three outcomes are highly correlated and should not be considered independent findings.

Significantly lower odds ratios were also observed for low birth weight among all births in the RW 2 and RW 3 groups and for very low birth weight in the RW 1 group. There was no indication of a pattern consistent with a decreasing or increasing dose-response relationship with reclaimed water for any of the outcomes.

Birth Defects. Overall, the results indicate that birth defects occur at about the same rate in the reclaimed water and control groups. The groups with lower percentages of reclaimed water (RW 1 and RW 2) tend to have higher rates than the control group, whereas the group with the highest percentage of reclaimed water (RW 4) tends to have rates similar to or lower than the control group. Six of the 76 odds ratios for specific birth defect categories indicated significantly higher rates in the reclaimed water groups than in the control group, and two indicated a significantly lower rate. The six higher odds ratios occurred as follows:

- RW 1: Neural tube defects; major cardiac defects; all other defects

- RW 2: Defects of the ears, eyes, face and neck; other digestive system defects

- RW 3: Limb defects.

The two significantly lower odds ratios occurred in the RW 1 group for defects of the integument and for chromosomal syndromes. Notably, RW 4, the group with the highest percentage of reclaimed water, exhibited no significantly higher or lower odds ratios for any birth defect category.

The results present no consistent evidence of a dose-response relationship between any birth defect and reclaimed water. For neural tube defects (NTDs), however, RW 1, RW 2, and RW 3 had relatively high odds ratios (1.52, 1.44, and 1.55, respectively), suggesting that there might be an increased risk of NTDs in these three groups compared with the control group. For 13 of the 19 birth defect categories, the rate in RW 4 is lower than the rate in RW 1. RW 4 has the highest rates for three categories: major cardiac defects, pyloric stenosis, and chromosomal syndromes. In these three defect categories, reclaimed water seems an unlikely explanation for this pattern of results for two reasons: all three odds ratios are relatively small (1.23, 1.09, and 1.13), indicating a weak association with reclaimed water, and the odds ratios for these outcomes in the other three reclaimed water groups do not follow a pattern consistent with a dose-response relationship. Thus, we conclude that this study did not find an association between reclaimed water and increased rates of birth defects.

INTERPRETATION OF STUDY RESULTS

Meaning of Null Effects

This epidemiologic study was unable to detect an association between adverse birth outcomes and reclaimed water or consistent evidence of a dose-response relationship. When such associations are not found in a study, the results are described as "null effects" or "null findings." Null effects may result when reclaimed water is truly not related to adverse birth outcomes, when sampling error makes the statistical estimates too imprecise to discern the true effects, or when it is impossible to control for potentially confounding factors that might bias the results. To understand what null effects mean, we must evaluate the precision of the estimates. We do this by considering the width of the confidence intervals and by determining the magnitude of effects that, in theory, could have been detected by this study. If the confidence intervals are narrow, meaning that we could detect small deviations from odds ratios of 1.0, this would indicate that any null findings reflect a truly null relationship rather than a lack of precision. It is more difficult to evaluate how potential confounders for which data are unavailable might affect the interpretation of the null effects.

In general, narrow confidence intervals indicate a precise estimate and a high level of certainty that null findings are not masking truly large effects. Wide confidence intervals allow for the possibility that we observe no statistically significant effects even though the true odds ratios are large. For most outcomes in this study, the odds ratios are less than 2.0 and the confidence intervals are relatively narrow with an upper bound substantially smaller than 2.0. For some outcomes, the confidence intervals are somewhat wider—notably, neural tube defects, limb defects, all other birth defects, and birth defect syndromes other than chromosomal. These outcomes are extremely rare, and hence the estimates are imprecise. For patent ductus arteriosus and cleft defects, the confidence intervals for some of the reclaimed water groups include values near or above 2.0. For these outcomes, the upper bound on the confidence interval is higher because the estimated odds ratios exceed 1.0 and the precision of these estimates is low. Most of the confidence intervals reported in Tables 4.4 through 4.9 are relatively narrow, demonstrating that the null findings of this study reflect truly null effects rather than too little precision to identify large effects.

We can further explore the meaning of the null effects by determining the minimum odds ratios that this study was likely to detect. The probability that a study will detect an effect if it truly exists (i.e., identify an odds ratio as "statistically significantly greater than 1.0" or "statistically significantly less than 1.0") is referred to as "power." For each outcome in the four reclaimed water study groups, we have estimated the size of the smallest effect (i.e., the minimum odds ratio) that could have been detected by the statistical test conducted with power of 80 percent (or probability 0.8). These minimum odds ratios are presented in Appendix D.

When a statistical test is significant (i.e., when the test statistic is extreme and unlikely to have occurred by chance when there is no effect), we are able to reject the null hypothesis of no effect in favor of the alternative hypothesis of an effect. By rejecting the null hypothesis only when we have extreme values of the test statistic, statistical tests minimize the chance of concluding that an effect exists when it does not. On the other hand, statistical tests can fail to reject the null hypothesis even if an effect exists. The less likely a test is to fail to reject the null hypothesis when an effect exists, the more powerful the test is.

The power of statistical tests depends on the size of the effect: the larger the effect, the smaller the risk of failing to reject the null hypothesis. Power also depends on the precision of the estimated test statistic and the sample size. More precise estimates yield tests with greater power. Larger samples increase the precision of the estimate and thus increase the power of the test.

Although the study detected few statistically significant results, it had statistical power to detect odds ratios equal to or greater than the minimum odds ratios given in Appendix D. For most outcomes, these minimum odds ratios indicate that the study has 80 percent power to detect odds ratios of a magnitude of 2.0 or less. This means that if the true rate of a particular adverse birth outcome were twice as high in one of the reclaimed water groups than in the control group, the study would be able to detect such a difference 80 percent of the time. For four of the less common outcomes (syndromes other than chromosomal, patent ductus arteriosus, cleft defects, and intestinal atresias), the minimum odds ratios are about 2.0. For the three least common outcomes (neural tube defects, limb defects, and "all other defects"), the minimum odds ratios are about 3.0. If study results indicate no effect (i.e., null effects), we can conclude only that the effect, if any, is most likely smaller than the minimum effect the study is capable of detecting. Therefore, for most outcomes, the study has sufficient power to detect effects of a magnitude that would be of concern.

Evaluating the Dose-Response Relationship

Based on the magnitude and pattern of results, we have concluded that this study does not provide evidence of a dose-response relationship between reclaimed water and any of the adverse birth outcomes. This conclusion is based on evidence that, for most outcomes in the study, the odds ratios for the four reclaimed water groups are close to 1.0 and do not increase in magnitude consistent with a dose-response relationship (i.e., OR(RW 1) < OR(RW 2) < OR(RW 3) < OR(RW 4)). Based on the analyses presented in this report and other results not presented,[2] we are confident in saying that the study does not provide empirical evidence of a dose-response relationship between reclaimed water and adverse birth outcomes. However, we must qualify that conclusion by stating that the study lacks precision for detecting a dose-response relationship.

Generalizability

A question arises regarding whether the findings of this study can be generalized to other situations. Because many areas throughout the United States are considering augmenting drinking water supplies with reclaimed water as a solution to increasingly scarce new water sources, issues related to the health effects of this practice have become important at the national level. There is interest in whether the results of this and other studies of the Montebello Forebay population can be extrapolated to populations in other geographic areas, as well as to the same population in different time periods and different situations.

---

[2]We fitted alternative models, such as the linear models, which would have provided some evidence of a dose-response relationship, if it existed.

The results of the studies of the Montebello Forebay population provide important information in the national debate, but should be interpreted cautiously. Before generalizing the results to other populations, one must consider the similarities and differences between the Montebello Forebay and the populations to which the results would be applied. It would be unwise to generalize to populations whose demographic and socioeconomic characteristics and exposure differ significantly from those in the Montebello Forebay. Even if the results are generalized to a similar populations (i.e., a largely urban, low- to middle-income, Hispanic population), the ability to infer is limited to the effects at the group level of serving reclaimed water. One cannot infer that individual exposure to reclaimed water has no effect, because this study was unable to measure individual exposure.

LIMITATIONS OF STUDY DESIGN

Lack of Information on Individual Exposure

Epidemiologic studies of water quality and health outcomes often explore the relationship between a particular chemical constituent of the water and adverse health outcomes. For example, Waller et al. (1998) compared levels of total and specific THMs and rates of spontaneous abortions. Because there is no evidence that reclaimed water contains higher levels of compounds known or suspected to cause adverse birth outcomes, we used the percentage of reclaimed water as a surrogate for the overall quality of the water. An alternative study design would have been to measure the association between particular adverse birth outcomes and the level of individual constituents in the water supplies containing reclaimed water. Almost all measured constituents are below the maximum contaminant level, leading to the conclusion that they should cause no health effects. Other constituents either cannot be or are not measured routinely. The cost of gathering data on the level of these substances would be prohibitive in the large number of water supplies in the Montebello Forebay.

Exposure to reclaimed water was estimated in this study as an annual average percentage at the ZIP code level. The percentage of reclaimed water in the water supplies of the Montebello Forebay was estimated for this study using a model based on hydrogeologic and statistical theory. Input to the model consisted of actual data on the operating parameters of the water systems serving residential customers. The results of the model were validated to the extent possible by Bookman-Edmonston, Inc. Nonetheless, the methods yield approximate measures, subject to some measurement error. In addition, exposure was estimated as an annual percentage, without considering the inevitable fluctuations of the percentage of reclaimed water served throughout the months of each year. Each birth record was assigned the percentage of reclaimed water served to the ZIP code of the mother's residence at the time of birth. In the analyses, the births were classified into one of four reclaimed water groups based on this percentage.

Information on exposure to reclaimed water is not available for individuals. The information on exposure is based on the percentage of reclaimed water in the water supply of each ZIP code rather than how much reclaimed water each individual consumes. Thus, many assumptions have to be met in order for the percentage of reclaimed water for the ZIP code to be an accurate measure of exposure for individual women in this study (Reif et al., 1996). These include the following conditions: the address recorded on the birth certificate represents the mother's residence during the entire pregnancy; the home water supply was not altered by a filtering system; most consumption (drinking and bathing) of water occurred at home; the mother drank tap water and not bottled water at home; the estimated percentage of reclaimed water in the ZIP code accurately represents the true percentage of reclaimed water in the tap water throughout the ZIP code (at least within the range of percentages represented by the group). Although some of these assumptions (e.g., use of water filters) might be rare enough to have little effect on the results, others (e.g., consumption of bottled water) might lead to substantial exposure misclassification and, therefore, yield results for individuals that differ from the results presented in this report.

Because we use a ZIP code–level, rather than an individual-level, measure of exposure, we are testing the hypothesis of an association between residence in an area with some percentage of reclaimed water in the drinking water supply and adverse birth outcomes. We are not testing for an association between individual consumption of reclaimed water and adverse birth outcomes. Because this study uses a ZIP code–level measure of exposure, the results may be subject to the bias associated with the ecologic fallacy problem. The ecologic fallacy arises when a conclusion regarding associations at the individual level are based on an analysis of group-level data. In ecologic studies, lack of information on exposure and outcome at the individual level leads to a situation in which the exposure status of an individual who develops a health outcome is unknown. The bias that may result from analyzing group-level data can affect the ecologic association, making it seem to be stronger or weaker than the true association at the individual level. In most studies, however, the bias increases the magnitude of the true association (Morgenstern, 1982).

Effect of Population Mobility

Change of residence during pregnancy might also result in misclassification of exposure (Reif et al., 1996). Based on 1990 census data, 51 percent of people living in the Montebello Forebay reported that they had lived in the same residence five years earlier (in 1985). In the control area, fewer (45 percent) had resided in the same place for five years or longer. One study of birth defects in California found that 25 percent of women moved one or more times during pregnancy (Shaw and Malcoe, 1991). These high mobility rates imply that many mothers in the study areas may have been exposed to more than one water supply during their pregnancy, of which perhaps only the water supply at the time of birth contained reclaimed water.

Information on the mobility of pregnant women in the study areas is not available. In general, women who live in the reclaimed water areas at the beginning of their pregnancy, but move out of these areas before giving birth, will be excluded from the analysis or possibly misclassified as to their exposure. Women who live elsewhere during the first part of their pregnancy and move into the reclaimed water areas toward the end of their pregnancy will be included in the analysis. Therefore, the movement out of the area will decrease the *number* of pregnant women who have been "exposed" to reclaimed water during the first trimester of pregnancy, the period during which fetal development is most susceptible to teratogens. As new residents move into the area to replace those who have moved out, the *proportion* of women who were "exposed" to reclaimed water during the first trimester of their pregnancies will also decrease. Although outmigration will not bias estimates of exposure effects (assuming outmigration is independent of outcome status), it reduces statistical power by reducing the sample size of exposed women (Hatch et al., 1990). The inclusion of women who recently moved into the area, however, will result in exposure misclassification and weaken estimates of effect (Polissar, 1980).

Inability to Control for Potentially Confounding Variables

In this study, the multiple regression methods controlled for differences between the reclaimed water and control groups in many important determinants of risk (i.e., risk factors) for these adverse birth outcomes (see model covariates in Table 3.4). However, we were not able to control for some important risk factors for which data are not available. The inability to control for maternal smoking, in particular, is problematic because it is known to be a strong risk factor for low birth weight infants. Other potentially confounding variables include clinical characteristics of the pregnancy, alcohol consumption, maternal occupation, and other environmental exposures. The study design assumes individuals with these confounding characteristics were distributed equally on average between the reclaimed water and control groups. If the distribution of these factors differs among the study groups, the observed pattern of results could be biased.

Effect of Spontaneous Abortions and Elective Terminations on Adverse Birth Outcomes

To fully understand these results, the reader should keep in mind that birth defects analyzed in this study are limited to those identified among infants who have survived the entire period of gestation and are born alive. The adverse birth outcomes among liveborn infants represent a subset of all adverse pregnancy outcomes, many of which render the developing fetus inviable, resulting in death prior to birth. Fetal deaths occurring early in pregnancy are called spontaneous abortions, whereas later in pregnancy they are called stillbirths or fetal deaths. Prenatal screening and elective termination of pregnancy have decreased the rate of selected birth defects (anencephaly, spina bifida, encephalocele, and Down's syndrome) among liveborn infants (Centers for Disease Control and Prevention, 1992; Yen et al., 1992, Cragan et al., 1995; Centers for Disease Control and Prevention, 1994). Birth defects and other adverse outcomes among liveborn infants are, therefore, a subset of adverse birth outcomes among all conceptions.

In this study, we assumed that the proportion of infants with a birth defect who survive the gestational period and are born alive does not differ between the reclaimed water and control groups. If this assumption is true, comparing the rates of birth defects among liveborn infants in the reclaimed water and control groups provides an unbiased estimate of the relative frequency of defects among all conceptions. Given that data on birth defects and other adverse outcomes are not readily available for all conceptions, but are available for all live births, limiting the study to the population of liveborn infants seems reasonable.

COMPARISON OF RESULTS WITH OTHER STUDIES

Previous Epidemiologic Studies of the Montebello Forebay

This study differs in several ways from the earlier epidemiologic studies of the Montebello Forebay (Frerichs et al., 1981, 1982, 1983). First, the 12-year period evaluated by the current study (1982–1993) is more recent than the period evaluated by previous studies (1969–1980). Second, the percentage of reclaimed water is higher in most Montebello Forebay water supplies during this period because the volume of reclaimed water used to recharge the groundwater basin increased markedly between 1980 and 1990. Third, the population receiving reclaimed water is almost twice the size of that studied in the earlier studies. This increase is explained primarily by the spread of reclaimed water in the groundwater basin and, consequently, additional water systems using groundwater containing reclaimed water. Two of these three factors—the higher percentage of reclaimed water and the much larger population—should increase the likelihood of finding an effect of reclaimed water on the health of those living in the area, if such an effect exists.

The epidemiologic studies of the Montebello Forebay populations completed in the early 1980s concluded that rates of adverse birth outcomes did not differ significantly between the areas receiving reclaimed water and the control areas (Frerichs et al., 1981, 1982, 1983). These studies analyzed rates of infant mortality, low birth weight, very low birth weight, and congenital malformations at the time of birth[3,4] based on vital statistics data from 1969 through 1980. Many aspects of the earlier studies differ from the current study, including the data sources, statistical methods, and control locations. Even so, the general conclusions are the same: Higher rates of adverse birth outcomes were not observed in populations receiving reclaimed water.

Another pattern worth noting is that the groups receiving lower percentages of reclaimed water have slightly higher rates of cancer, mortality, infectious disease (Sloss et al., 1996), and adverse birth outcomes. Although this pattern does not support an association between reclaimed water and any of these outcomes, the pattern may indicate that some aspect of the residential location or a characteristic of the population is responsible for the elevated rates in areas with less reclaimed water. Further investigation of the reasons for the higher rates may be indicated.

---

[3]Birth defects were analyzed for the years 1969–1971 in the earlier studies (Frerichs et al., 1981, 1982, 1983).

[4]The analysis in these earlier studies is based on birth defects diagnosed at the time of birth and recorded on the birth certificate. Because many birth defects are diagnosed after the infant leaves the hospital, these studies included only a subset of all defects. The current study derives its information on birth defects from an active surveillance system that includes all defects diagnosed during the first year of life. It therefore may be a better measure of the underlying rate of birth defects.

Epidemiologic Studies of Drinking Water and Adverse Birth Outcomes

As noted in Chapter Two, previous epidemiologic studies have found associations between specific drinking water constituents or particular sources of drinking water and higher rates of adverse birth outcomes. None of these previous studies focused on areas that intentionally reused reclaimed water (with the exception of those discussed in the section above). Several epidemiologic studies have suggested an association between drinking water and spontaneous abortion (Aschengrau et al., 1989; Swan et al., 1998; Waller et al., 1998). Others have reported higher rates of birth defects in areas with soft water (Penrose, 1957; Lowe, 1971), industrially contaminated drinking water (Lagakos et al., 1986; Deane et al., 1989; Goldberg et al., 1990; Bove et al., 1995), water with differing levels of trace elements or minerals (Zierler et al., 1988; Aschengrau et al., 1993), and water with high nitrate levels (Dorsch et al., 1984; Scragg et al., 1982). The results of the current study do not indicate an association between the percentage of reclaimed water in the drinking water supply and any of the adverse birth outcomes examined (low and very low birth weight, preterm birth, infant mortality, or birth defects). Although other studies have found associations between specific constituents of drinking water and increased rates of adverse birth outcomes, this study did not test for associations with any specific constituents and, therefore, does not add information to this body of research.

STRENGTHS OF STUDY DESIGN

Quality of Outcome Data

In this study, the prenatal development measures were derived from vital statistics data for the State of California. Each birth or death certificate contains information about an event that has been registered with the vital statistics system. Birth weight, gestational age, and selected characteristics of the mother are also recorded on the birth certificate for a high percentage of births. These data are collected on a routine basis and are defined and recorded in a consistent manner. In addition, these health outcomes are ascertained in the same way for the entire population. Registration of births and deaths is virtually 100 percent complete in the United States. Some data elements (e.g., the ZIP code of residence at the time of birth and gestational age) may not be accurately recorded on the birth certificate. In this study, we must assume that no systematic difference exists between the study groups in the quality of the information.

Data on birth defects were obtained from the California Birth Defects Monitoring Program (CBDMP). The CBDMP collects and compiles information about birth defects diagnosed during the first year of life for infants in selected California counties (Stierman, 1994). The CBDMP uses active surveillance methods to record and track birth defects. Trained CBDMP staff collect data from hospitals, genetic clinics, and chromosome laboratories. Many records at these medical facilities are reviewed and evaluated to make sure a large percentage of diagnosed birth defects are identified. These methods are essential for obtaining an accurate and unbiased estimate of the frequency of birth defects in a population. As with vital records, the information on birth defects is recorded in a prescribed manner, resulting in consistent reporting across all study groups.

Other Strengths

If the results of this study are interpreted cautiously, it has several strengths. First, we were able to examine data for an extremely large population—452,275 infants born in selected areas of Los Angeles County over a 12-year period. Second, we were able to investigate a large number of health outcomes: Four outcomes related to prenatal development, infant mortality, and 19 categories of birth defects. Third, this study design allowed us to address the important policy question of whether women living in areas receiving reclaimed water are experiencing higher rates of adverse birth outcomes. Finally, because this study relied on existing data, its cost was moderate.

CONCLUSIONS

This epidemiologic study concludes that during the 12-year period from 1982–1993, the rates of adverse birth outcomes are similar in the Montebello Forebay region receiving reclaimed water and a control group not receiving any reclaimed water. Rates of these health outcomes are similar in groups receiving higher and lower percentages of reclaimed water. The analysis includes routinely collected data on low birth weight, very low birth weight, preterm birth, infant mortality, and 19 categories of birth defects. Some outcome rates were significantly higher and others were significantly lower for the reclaimed water groups than for the control group. In general, women living in areas with higher percentages of reclaimed water in their water supplies did not give birth to infants who have higher rates of adverse outcomes than women living in areas with lower percentages of reclaimed water.

The limitations of epidemiologic methods make drawing conclusions about the effects of reclaimed water on adverse birth outcomes difficult. In this study, we had no data on individual exposure to reclaimed water. The percentage of reclaimed water may not represent individual exposure accurately because of time spent away from home and consumption of bottled water and other beverages. In addition, personal characteristics that might affect the outcomes in this report—such as cigarette smoking, alcohol consumption, and occupational exposure—were assumed to be equal in the reclaimed water and control groups, but we could not control these in the analysis. If the distribution of these factors differs substantially between the reclaimed water and control groups, the pattern of results may be attributable to these differences or to other uncontrolled factors. Finally, the high population mobility in Los Angeles County could hamper detecting an effect. Despite the study's limitations, the patterns of results observed provide no evidence of an association between reclaimed water and adverse birth outcomes. The results of this or any other epidemiologic study cannot certify that reclaimed water has no effect on human health. We can conclude, however, that if reclaimed water is causing higher rates of any of these adverse birth outcomes, the increased risk is likely to be small.

FUTURE RESEARCH

This epidemiologic assessment compares rates of adverse birth outcomes in four groups receiving increasing percentages of reclaimed water with those in a control group not receiving any reclaimed water. Several important questions related to the health effects of reclaimed water, however, remain unanswered. First, how do other risk factors (e.g., smoking, alcohol consumption, occupational exposures) that might affect the rate of cancer, death, infectious disease, and adverse birth outcomes compare in the reclaimed water and control groups? Second, does individual exposure to reclaimed water (i.e., consumption of home tap water) differ between the reclaimed water and control groups? Studying these two questions would address some of the limitations of the design of this and the previous study of cancer incidence, mortality, and infectious disease (Sloss et al., 1996). Third, are rates of spontaneous abortions and infertility similar in the reclaimed water and control groups? Information on these outcomes would address important questions remaining about the association between reclaimed water and health outcomes.

EPIDEMIOLOGIC STUDIES OF DRINKING WATER AND ADVERSE BIRTH OUTCOMES

Table A.1

Summary of Studies of Drinking Water and Adverse Birth Outcomes

Authors, Outcome, and Population	Measure of Exposure	Results
Arbuckle et al., 1988. 130 cases of infants with central nervous system (CNS) malformations (ICD-8 740.0–743.9, ICD-9 740.0–742.9) identified by a registry; controls selected randomly from live birth files and matched (2:1) for county of maternal residence and date of birth; cases and controls drawn from all births in New Brunswick, Canada, 1973–1983.	Nitrate, chloride, and sulfate concentrations measured in drinking water samples taken after 1983 at addresses mentioned on birth or stillbirth records as maternal residence.	Exposure to increased nitrate levels (26 ppm) in private well water was associated with increased risk for CNS defects among children (RR = 2.30 (95% CI 0.73–7.29)).
Aschengrau et al., 1989. 286 cases of spontaneous abortion (< 27 weeks gestation) and 1,391 controls who delivered within one week of each case's pregnancy loss selected randomly among all women admitted to two hospitals in Boston, Massachusetts, July 1976–February 1978.	Routine analysis results for trace elements, metals, and hardness of public tap water in each subject's community. Exposure determined from water samples matched to the time of pregnancy and the conception date as close as possible for each pregnancy.	Increased incidence of spontaneous abortion associated with detectable levels of mercury; high levels of arsenic, potassium, and silica; moderately hard water; and surface water. Decreases were noted for high levels of alkalinity and sulfate as well as any level of nitrate.

Table A.1—continued

Authors, Outcome, and Population	Measure of Exposure	Results
Aschengrau et al., 1993. 1,039 congenital anomaly cases, 77 stillbirth cases, 55 neonatal death cases, and 1,177 controls born August 1977 through March 1980 at Brigham and Women's Hospital in Massachusetts.	Local water quality data collected routinely by a city or town was matched to each woman's address of residency at the time of pregnancy outcome or during the first trimester. Trace element levels, water source, and treatment mode (chlorination vs. chloramination) were collected for the public water supplies in (155) communities using the samples drawn closest to the conception date.	The frequency of stillbirths was increased for women exposed to chlorinated surface water (OR 2.6; 95% CI 0.9–7.5) and for women exposed to detectable lead levels (OR 2.1; 95% CI 0.6–7.2); the frequency of cardiovascular defects was increased relative to detectable lead levels (OR 2.2, 95% CI 0.9–5.7); the frequency of CNS defects was increased relative to the highest tertile of potassium (OR 6.3, 95% CI 1.1–37.3). The frequency of ear, face, and neck anomalies was increased in relation to detectable silver levels (OR 3.3, 95% CI 0.9–12.2), but the frequency decreased relative to high potassium levels (OR 0.2, 95% CI 0.1–0.7). The frequency of neonatal deaths was decreased relative to detectable fluoride levels (OR 0.4, 95% CI 0.2–1.0), and the frequency of musculoskeletal defects was decreased relative to detectable chromium levels (OR 0.4, 95% CI 0.2–1.0).
Bound et al., 1981. All (73,561) live births, stillbirths, and neonatal deaths occurring in Fylde of Lancashire, U.K, between 1956 and 1976 were examined for anencephalus as identified by medical officers of health.	Chemical analysis of drinking water to determine total water hardness in N. Fylde vs. S. Fylde; averages from 12 annual samples taken at two sampling points were used to calculate summer and winter exposure for each year between 1956 and 1976.	From 1957 to 1961 the incidence in N. Fylde was 4.4 per 1,000 births, compared to 1.8 cases per 1,000 births in S. Fylde. During this time both areas had soft water. From 1962 to 1969, overall incidence decreased to 1.8 cases per 1,000 births, and water quality changed to the slightly hard category.
Bove et al., 1995. All (80,938) live births and fetal deaths (594) between 1985 and 1988 for residents in 75 selected towns in northern New Jersey served by public water system and for which most births occurred within the state; information obtained from vital records and a (passive) birth defect registry; study outcomes were fetal death, low birth weight, various birth defects, and small size for gestational age.	Monthly estimates of source water contaminants from 1985 to 1988 assigned to gestational month of each live birth and fetal death. At a minimum, one tap water sample for each six-month interval was required for total trihalomethanes (TTHM), trichloroethylene, tetrachloroethylene, 1,1,1-trichloroethane, carbon tetrachloride, 1,2-dichloroethane, and benzene.	TTHM was associated with small size for gestational age (SGA), CNS defects, neural tube defects (NTD), oral clefts, and major cardiac defects (MCD). Carbon tetrachloride was associated with low birth weight, SGA, CNS defects, oral clefts, and NTD; trichloroethylene with CNS, NTD, and oral cleft; benzene with NTD and MCDs; 1,2-dichloroethane with MCDs.

Table A.1—continued

Authors, Outcome, and Population	Measure of Exposure	Results
Cohn et al., 1994. Birth defects, low birth weight, and small for gestational age among 80,000 births and fetal deaths in a 75-town region of New Jersey, 1985–1988.	Exposure to drinking water contamination estimated by monitoring data for drinking water systems in municipality of maternal residence at the time of birth or fetal death. Analysis included THMs and chlorinated solvents.	Positive associations between drinking water exposures and adverse reproductive outcomes. Exposure to >80 µg/l THMs resulted in increased odds for all birth defects (OR 1.6, 95% CI 1.2–2.1), NTDs (OR 3.0, 95% CI 1.2–7.1), low birth weight (OR 1.3, 95% CI 1.1–1.6), and small size for gestational age (OR 1.2, 95% CI 1.1–1.3). Exposure to PCE > 10 µg/l resulted in a significant increase in oral clefts (OR 3.5, 95% CI 1.3–9.7).
Deane et al., 1989. Pregnant women in two census tracts (exposed and not exposed) reported spontaneous abortion, birth defects, and low birth weight; Santa Clara County, California, residents during the entire pregnancy; January 1, 1980, through December 31, 1981.	Residence in area exposed to trichloroethane contaminated water (i.e., a single exposed census tract); maternal consumption of tap water assessed via telephone interviews.	The risk ratio (RR) for spontaneous abortion occurring in the exposed census tract was 2.3 (95% CI 1.3–4.2); for malformations, RR was 3.1 (95% CI 1.1–10.4); for spontaneous abortion and cold tap water consumption, RR was 2.1 (95% CI 1.3–3.5). No associations were found for either exposure and low birth weight.
Deane et al., 1992 (reanalysis of 1989 study). Same study population and outcomes as Deane et al., 1989.	Cold tap water consumption during pregnancy and three months prior to pregnancy among women living in two census tracts, one in which well water had been contaminated with trichloroethane; ascertained in telephone interview.	RR for spontaneous abortion and consumption of tap water was 3.4 (95% CI 0.6–19.40); for congenital abnormalities RR was 1.3 (95% CI 0.2–8.2). Increases for outcomes extended outside of the contamination area, so authors concluded that results not due to contamination event.
Dorsch et al., 1984 (and Scragg et al., 1982). 218 cases of congenital malformations; matched 1:1 with controls on hospital, maternal age, parity, and date of birth; identified from hospital delivery registers; rural South Australia; 1951–1979.	Groundwater vs. rainwater as drinking water source and nitrate levels in groundwater at the time of pregnancy obtained from local water authorities.	RR associated with maternal ground vs. rain water consumption was 2.8 (95% CI 1.9–5.1). The risk from groundwater consumption was high for CNS defects (RR = 3.5) and musculoskeletal defects (RR = 2.9). RRs for all anomalies increased with nitrate levels found in government bores (RR = 2.6 for 5–15 ppm, RR = 4.1 for >15 ppm of nitrate).
Elwood and Coldman, 1981. 468 fatal cases of anencephalus identified from death registration records and 4,129 randomly selected live births from the same localities (N = 142) as the cases with population >10,000; Canada; 1969–1972.	Data on 14 trace elements in drinking water were obtained from each locality; samples were collected between June 1970 and December 1972; the average for at least three water samples was applied to all births within that locality.	No significant association with any trace element after adjusting for demographic factors.

Table A.1—continued

Authors, Outcome, and Population	Measure of Exposure	Results
Fenster et al., 1992. 100 cases of spontaneous abortion (<20 weeks) identified by hospital pathology reports and 200 pregnant controls matched by time of last menstrual period and facility obtained from OB appointment logs at 2 Kaiser facilities; Santa Clara County, California, February–July 1987.	Following a water contamination incident involving trichloroethane, maternal consumption of tap and bottled water during the first 20 weeks of pregnancy was assessed via two computer-assisted telephone interviews at 24 weeks after last menstrual period and again at 48 weeks after last menstrual period.	Neither an increased risk from tap water consumption (OR = 0.71) nor a protective effect from bottled water was observed (OR = 1.10).
Fielding and Smithells, 1971. 132,900 births analyzed for incidence of anencephalus in three cities in England and Wales, 1963–1970.	Water hardness as measured annually for the three cities.	In southwest Lancashire (soft water) the incidence of anencephalus, was lower (2.9) than in two other cities with hard water (3.5). However, the introduction of a water-softening plant did not change the incidence of anencephalus in one of the cities with formerly hard water.
Goldberg et al., 1990. All cases of congenital cardiac disease (N = 707) identified from pediatric cardiology records born to parents living in Tucson Valley, Arizona, between January 1, 1969, and December 31, 1987.	Parents were considered exposed if they resided or worked in an area of well water contamination with trichloroethylene for one month prior to and during the first trimester of pregnancy.	The risk of having a child with a congenital heart disease was three times higher for parents exposed to contaminated well water than for unexposed parents. The rate of congenital heart disease decreased for exposed residents.
Hertz-Picciotto et al., 1989. 470 cases of spontaneous abortion (<28 weeks) and 1,239 randomly sampled controls selected from a cohort of recognized pregnancies at three Kaiser facilities; the cohort had been established previously to investigate malathion exposure; Santa Clara County, California, July 1, 1981–March 30, 1982.	Maternal consumption of tap and bottled water during pregnancy was assessed; distinguished between tap water source as groundwater, surface water, or mixture of both.	Hazard ratio for spontaneous abortion of 1.5, 95% CI (1.1–2.0) for tap water consumption. Tap water consumed from a groundwater source was associated with the greatest risk (hazard ratio of 1.7). However, no reproductive toxins were identified in the water source and inconsistencies in the reporting suggested recall bias.
Klotz et al., 1999. Statewide case-control study of NTDs and selected drinking water contaminants in New Jersey population, 1993–1994.	Exposure based on public monitoring records for fourth week of gestation and tap water samples one year later.	Association between THMs in drinking water and NTDs, and chlorine residuals and NTDs.

Table A.1—continued

Authors, Outcome, and Population	Measure of Exposure	Results
Kramer et al., 1992. 159 low birth weight infants (<2,500 g), 342 premature infants (<37 weeks), and 187 growth-retarded infants (<5th percentile of weight for gestational age); matched 5:1 for maternal age, parity, education, marital status, smoking, and prenatal care; identified from birth certificates of infants born to white women in towns that obtained drinking water from a single source and with a population of 1,000–5,000; Iowa, January 1, 1989, to June 30, 1990.	Exposures of chloroform, dichlorobromomethane, dibromochloromethane, and bromoform assessed ecologically according to maternal residence at time of birth and data from a 1987 municipal water survey.	Residence in municipalities with chloroform concentrations $\geq$ 10 mg/L showed increased risk for intrauterine growth retardation; OR = 1.8; 95% CI (1.1–2.9).
Lagakos et al., 1986. 4,396 pregnancies that terminated in Woburn, Massachusetts, between 1960 and 1982 identified from a random sample of 5,010 households who resided in Woburn prior to 1979; outcomes were spontaneous abortion, perinatal death, low birth weight, 14 categories of birth defects; outcome data was obtained in a 1982 telephone survey.	Estimates of annual exposure to several chlorinated organics (trichloroethylene, tetra-chloroethylene, and chloroform) in drinking water drawn from contaminated wells between October 1964 and May 1979; estimates were based on a detailed model of regional and temporal distribution of waters from the contaminated wells. Time dependent estimates assigned to each pregnancy based on maternal residence in the year the pregnancy ended.	Contaminated water consumption was associated with perinatal death after 1970 and contributed to eye/ear defects and CNS/oral cleft anomalies. No association was found for low birth weight or spontaneous abortions.
Lowe et al., 1971. Deaths from perinatal anencephalus among 92,982 live and stillborn infants of residents in 58 county boroughs in England and Wales between 1963 and 1967.	Water content and calcium content for county boroughs with total populations >00,000 in 1961 from published sources of local water authorities.	Inverse relationship between frequency of perinatal mortality due to anencephalus and total water hardness (r = –0.220) and calcium content (r = –0.289).
Morton et al., 1976. 48 local authority areas analyzed for incidence of congenital nervous system defects; used malformation rates previously published by Lowe et al., South Wales, 1964–1966.	Concentrations of 20 trace elements in domestic water supply measured for each of the 48 areas studied; water was sampled morning and evening on one day in July 1973. At least 15 pairs of samples were obtained within each area.	Significant positive association with aluminum. Significant negative association found for calcium, barium, and copper. The associations with barium and copper were the strongest.

Table A.1—continued

Authors, Outcome, and Population	Measure of Exposure	Results
Savitz, et al., 1995. Medically treated cases of miscarriage (126), preterm deliveries (<37 weeks) (244), and low birth weight (<2,500g) (178) delivered in Orange and Durham County, North Carolina, September 1988 to August 1989. Controls were selected as the next non-case and same race baby delivered in the same hospital (1:1 matching).	Telephone interviews with mothers elicited the drinking water source and amount during pregnancy; and THM concentrations during pregnancy were estimated from documents of five public water supply companies servicing the area; quarterly THM averages closest to the fourth week of gestation for the miscarriages and closest to the 28th week of gestation for all other outcomes were used to determine exposure.	Water source was not related to any of the studied pregnancy outcomes. THM concentration and dose (concentration × amount) were not related to pregnancy outcome, with the possible exception of an increased risk of miscarriage in the highest sextile of THM concentration (adjusted odds ratio = 2.8, 95% confidence interval = 1.1–2.7), which was not part of an overall dose-response gradient.
Shaw et al., 1990. 145 cases of severe cardiac anomaly diagnosed during the first year of life by a state birth defect monitoring system and 176 controls randomly selected from vital statistics files of all live births in Santa Clara County, California, births between January 1981 and December 1983.	Residence in area with water contamination incident involving trichloroethane; maternal tap water consumption as well as dermal and inhalation exposure was assessed via telephone interviews; water source identified by address where mother resided or worked during the first trimester.	A positive association was found between consumption of >4 glasses of home tap water per day during first trimester and cardiac anomaly in child (OR = 2.0, 95% CI 1.0–4.0). Negative association found between consumption of bottled water during pregnancy and cardiac anomaly (OR = 0.04, 95% CI 0.002–0.64).
St. Leger et al., 1980. 108 cases of neural tube malformations; matched 1:1 with controls on sex, date of birth, maternal age and social class; all births within Cardiff identified by Cardiff Birth Survey; Cardiff, Wales *(note: no years given)*.	Water concentrations of 11 trace elements and hardness from tap water sampled from each dwelling over a non-specified, two-year period.	A statistically significant mean difference between cases and controls was found only for zinc (–0.059 ppm, 95% CI (–0.104—0.014); authors concluded that tap water was unlikely to be of relevance for NTDs in Cardiff.
Swan et al., 1989. 106 cases of cardiac anomaly (ICD-9 745.0 –747.9) identified by a registry compared to a random sample of all live births among residents of Santa Clara County, California, January 1981–December 1983.	Maternal residence (or work location) in area served by water contaminated with trichloroethane; an exposure gradient across the exposed area was derived from detailed hydrogeologic analysis. Tap water consumption during the first trimester was assessed by retrospective telephone interview.	During the exposed time period an increased risk for cardiac anomaly within the exposed area was found (RR = 2.2, 95% CI 1.2–4.0). No increased risk was observed during the unexposed time window. However, the observed spatial distribution of cases was not concurrent with the gradient of exposure determined by hydrogeologic modeling.

Table A.1—continued

Authors, Outcome, and Population	Measure of Exposure	Results
Swan et al., 1998. 5,342 pregnant women in 1990–1991 in prepaid medical plan from three California counties; pregnancy outcomes (spontaneous abortion or stillbirth) from hospital/medical records (91%) or interview, questionnaire or birth certificate.	Region I = groundwater and surface water mixture in northern California, Region II = mostly surface water in northern California, Region III = groundwater only in southern California; number of glasses of home tap water and bottled water from interview (cold, heated, straight from tap, standing, refrigerated, filter/purifier used).	Strong association between tap water consumption and spontaneous abortion in Region I only; high consumption of cold tap water compared with none (OR = 2.2, 95% CI = 1.2–3.9); high consumption of tap water and no bottled water compared to high consumption of bottled water and no tap water (OR = 4.6, 95% CI = 2.0–10.6).
Waller et al., 1998. Prospective study of 5,342 pregnant women in prepaid health plan; pregnancy outcomes (spontaneous abortion or stillbirth) ascertained from hospital or medical records (91%) or through interview or birth certificate; 5,144 available for analysis.	Detailed information on consumption of home tap water through telephone interview; level of TTHMs and four individual THMs based on average measurements by utility during first trimester.	Women reporting more than 5 glasses per day of cold tap water containing 75 or more μg per liter TTHM had OR of 1.8 for spontaneous abortion (SA) (95% CI = 1.1–3.0); only one of four THMs (bromodichloromethane) was associated with SA (OR = 2.0; 95% CI = 1.2–3.5).
Windham et al., 1992. 626 cases of spontaneous abortion (<20 weeks) and 1,300 controls; matched 2:1 on last menstrual period and hospital of birth; selected from medical records and live births at the same hospital, respectively; Santa Clara County, California, January 1986–February 1987.	Average consumption of cold tap water and bottled water during first trimester of pregnancy ascertained in telephone interviews.	Crude Odds Ratio (COR) for any vs. no tap water—1.2 (95% CI 1.0–1.5) with no dose-response effect. COR for any vs. no bottled water—0.79 (95% CI 0.65–0.96) with an inverse dose-response effect.
Wrensch et al., 1992. Expansion of the study of Deane, et al., 1989, to four study areas in Santa Clara County; pregnancies between 1980 and 1985 for which the woman resided in the same area for entire pregnancy. Pregnancies enumerated in 1986 from household survey. Outcomes included spontaneous abortion, low birth weight and birth defects.	Number of glasses of cold tap water and bottled water consumed during pregnancy and three months prior assessed via structured telephone interview.	Increased risk for spontaneous abortion and any vs. no tap water (OR = 6.9, 95% CI 2.7–17.7); decreased risk for spontaneous abortion and any vs. no bottled water (OR = 0.26, 95% CI 0.16–0.43); no association between low birth weight and either tap or bottle water.

Table A.1—continued

Authors, Outcome, and Population	Measure of Exposure	Results
Zierler et al., 1988. 207 cases of congenital heart disease and 655 randomly sampled controls born during the same year as the case; cases identified from birth defect registry and controls from birth certificates living in Massachusetts communities with public drinking water supplies, April 1, 1980, to March 31, 1983.	Contaminant levels in maternal drinking water from samples drawn closest to date of conception; interval from date of sample to date of conception ranged from 0 to 1,190 days, with a mean of 227 days. For 80% of the subjects the contaminant levels had been measured within one year of conception.	No chemical increased the frequency of congenital heart disease overall; detectable amounts of selenium were associated with significantly less congenital heart disease; any detectable amounts of arsenic were associated with a threefold increase in occurrence of coarctation of the aorta; mercury and lead were associated with a 60–80% increase in patent ductus arteriosus.

METHODS USED TO ESTIMATE THE PERCENTAGE OF RECLAIMED WATER IN MONTEBELLO FOREBAY GROUNDWATER SUPPLIES

The following description of the four methods used to estimate the percentage of reclaimed water in the Montebello Forebay groundwater supplies is based on the report by Bookman-Edmonston Engineering, Inc. (1993). They were direct calculation from a sulfate ion model (Nellor et al., 1984), regression analysis (Weisberg, 1985), the Kriging analytic method (Davis and McCullaugh, 1975), and an analysis of travel time contours (similar to the sulfate ion method described in Nellor et al., 1984).

SULFATE ION MODELING

The first method used to estimate reclaimed water in the groundwater supply was sulfate ion modeling, a method that uses the sulfate ion as a tracer for groundwater movement. The theory behind this method is that the sulfate concentration in the Colorado River water (a water source used since 1954 to replenish the Montebello Forebay groundwater basin) is substantially higher than the sulfate concentrations of the other types of water in the groundwater basin: storm water, native groundwater, and reclaimed water. Sulfate is considered a conservative material, the concentration of which is not likely to be affected by either vertical or horizontal movement through soil. Therefore, the sulfate concentration in groundwater pumped from the Montebello Forebay basin was used to estimate the relative proportion of Colorado River water in the groundwater. Any increase in the sulfate concentration at a particular location is indicative of the increased presence of Colorado River water.

In contrast, reclaimed water is not so easily identifiable because of its heterogeneous minerals composition. Because both waters are recharged in the same spreading basins, the relative proportion of reclaimed water in water pumped from a given service area in the groundwater basin can be estimated for any given year from the percentage of Colorado River water derived from sulfate measurements. This method assumes that both types of water follow a similar movement pattern in the groundwater basin. An empirical model was used to derive Colorado River "replacement values," which represent the percentage of native groundwater that has been replaced with Colorado River water through the process of replenishment.

The replacement value for a given well in a given year can be calculated using the following equation:

$$R_c = \frac{1}{x} \times \frac{(W_s - G_s)}{(C_s - G_s)} \times 100,$$

where R_c = percentage replacement of native groundwater with Colorado River water,

W_s = sulfate concentration of a well

G_s = sulfate concentration of native groundwater (assumed constant)

C_s = sulfate concentration of Colorado River water (assumed constant)

x = dilution factor.

The dilution factor represents the percentage of Colorado River water in the water used to recharge the Montebello Forebay in any given year. Annual dilution factors were calculated for the years 1954 to 1974 and were found to have no significant effect on the percentage replacement values. Replacement values for reclaimed water were obtained by shifting replacement values for sulfate by eight years. The eight-year time lag accounts for the difference between the year Colorado River water was first spread (1954) and the year reclaimed water was first spread (1962). The method assumes that the flow of reclaimed water follows the same groundwater dynamics as the flow of Colorado River water, lagged by eight years. This procedure can be represented as

$$R_r(1962) = R_c(1954)$$

where R_r = percentage replacement for reclaimed water

R_c = percentage replacement for Colorado River water.

Finally, the replacement value for reclaimed water was multiplied by the proportional factor F to account for the percentage of reclaimed water in the water used to recharge the basin. Proportional factors were also shifted to account for a time lag between spreading and arrival of reclaimed water at a particular well. Assuming that it takes one year for reclaimed water to reach a particular well, the corresponding proportional factor (F) would be shifted by one year. For example,

$$R_r'(1963) = R_r(1963) \times F(1962)$$

These time values were determined on the basis of the lag between the first spreading of Colorado River water for recharge and the first appearance of sulfate in a particular well. The proportion of reclaimed water in the groundwater supply of a service area is then calculated by summing the volume of reclaimed water in all wells in a service area and dividing it by the total volume of water in a service area. For example, for 1963:

$$P_r(1963) = \frac{\sum [R_{ri}(1963) \times AFY_i(1963)]}{\sum AFY_i(1963)}$$

where P_r =   percentage water pumped that is reclaimed

   R_{ri} =   replacement value for reclaimed water for i^{th} well

   AFY_i =   total water production for i^{th} well.

The sulfate modeling technique could not be used after 1982, because the use of Colorado River water for groundwater recharge in the Montebello Forebay ended in 1974. The eight-year time lag between the spreading of Colorado River water and reclaimed water allowed the use of Colorado River water replacement values for the years preceding 1974 to determine reclaimed water replacement values, and the percentages of reclaimed water in groundwater, until 1982. However, after 1982 the sulfate model was used only to a very limited extent. Instead, one of three other analytical methods was employed to derive the annual percentage of reclaimed water in the Montebello Forebay groundwater supplies for the years from 1983 to 1991.

Eventually, the process of groundwater recharge completely replaces the native groundwater. For those wells with 100 percent groundwater replacement prior to 1974, the proportion of reclaimed water in groundwater in any given year was assumed to be equal to the proportion of reclaimed water in the recharge sources X years earlier, where X is the lag time for that well.

REGRESSION ANALYSIS

For the period 1983 to 1991, regression analysis was used to estimate the percentage of reclaimed water for most of the water systems. Using regression methods, the volume of reclaimed water in the groundwater was correlated with the volume of reclaimed water spread based on annual data for 1960 to 1982. If a correlation of 0.80 or greater was found between the volume of reclaimed water in groundwater and the volume of reclaimed water spread in any given year, the regression model was used to predict the percentage of reclaimed water for the water systems for the years 1983 to 1990. If the correlation from the regression was less than 0.80, one of the two remaining techniques was used to estimate the annual percentage of reclaimed water in the groundwater supply.

KRIGING METHOD

For water systems with a correlation of less than 0.80 in the regression analysis, the statistical Kriging technique was used to estimate the percentage of reclaimed water. The Kriging technique assumes that spatial proximity will lead to a high correlation of some parameters. In this case, the assumption was that spatial proximity of two wells would lead to a high correlation between the percentages of reclaimed water in the pumped groundwater from the two wells. Based on this assumption, Bookman-Edmonston Engineering, Inc., used data from wells with known reclaimed water percentages to estimate the percentage of reclaimed water in groundwater pumped from neighboring wells.

TRAVEL TIME CONTOUR METHOD

The travel time contour method was employed to estimate the time required for water to travel from the spreading basin to a particular well in the Montebello Forebay (i.e., "travel time"). This method was used for water systems that had a correlation of less than 0.80 in the regression analysis and were too far from other wells to use the Kriging technique. It was also used for those few instances when the results from the sulfate-ion method provided clearly erroneous results. It is believed these occurred because of higher-than-normal background sulfate levels, which indicated the arrival of Colorado River recharge water when, in fact, none had yet reached the well in question. This method entailed using a map of the Montebello Forebay showing travel time contours for wells for which this information was known. From these maps, the travel time could be estimated for wells in the region with unknown travel times. The travel time was then used to estimate the percentage of reclaimed water in the groundwater supply by applying values for wells on the same contour.

PERCENTAGE OF RECLAIMED WATER IN MONTEBELLO FOREBAY WATER SYSTEM SERVICE AREAS AND ZIP CODES BY YEAR, 1982–1993

This appendix contains information on the percentage of reclaimed water received by the Montebello Forebay region during the period of this study. Table C.1 lists the names and an identifying number for each of the water systems in the Montebello Forebay region. Table C.2 presents the estimated annual percentages of reclaimed water for each water system service area, listed by identifying number. The percentages in Table C.2 were generated by the staff of Bookman-Edmonston Engineering, Inc., using the methods described in Appendix B. (The letters A, B, C, etc., following the system number in Table C.2 denote service areas within the water systems listed in Table C.1. These service areas are shown on the water system map of the Montebello Forebay (available on request).) Table C.3 presents annual percentages of reclaimed water for each ZIP code in the Montebello Forebay region estimated for this study using the methods described in Chapter Three. Figure C.1 shows a series of line graphs, each of which represents one ZIP code in the Montebello Forebay region. Each graph shows one or more lines, each of which represents the percentage of reclaimed water annually from 1981 to 1993 for a water system service area within the ZIP code. The bold line on each graph represents the weighted average of the individual service areas within the ZIP code. We used this weighted average in the analyses as the exposure measure for births occurring in the ZIP code.

Table C.1

**Numbers and Names of Montebello
Forebay Water Systems**

Water System Number	Name of Water System
1	California Water Service Company
3	City of Downey
5	City of Commerce
6	La Habra Heights County Water District
7	Mutual Water Owners Association of Los Nietos
8	City of Montebello
9	Montebello Land and Water Company
10	City of Norwalk
11	Orchard Dale County Water District
12	Park Water Company
13	Pico County Water District
14	City of Pico Rivera
15	San Gabriel Valley Water Company
16	City of Santa Fe Springs
17	South Montebello Irrigation District
18	Southern California Water Company
19	Southwest Suburban Water Company
20	City of Whittier
24	City of Lynwood
25	Maywood Mutual Water Company No. 3
26	Peerless Land and Water Company
28	Rancho Los Amigos
30	City of South Gate
31	Tract No. 180 Mutual Water Company
32	Tract No. 349 Mutual Water Company
33	Bellflower-Somerset Mutual Water Company
34	City of Huntington Park
35	City of Paramount
36	Bellflower Home Garden
37	Bigby Townsite
39	County Water Co.
43	Maywood No. 1
44	Maywood No. 2
46	Walnut Park Mutual Water Company
47	Beverly Acres Mutual Water Users Association
48	Industry Water Works
49	Los Angeles Department of Water and Power
50	City of Vernon

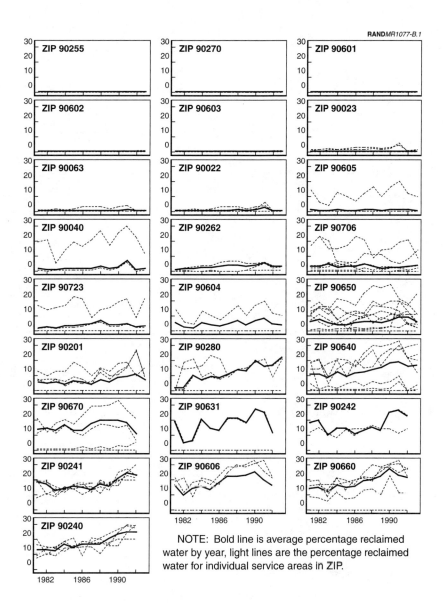

RAND*MR1077-B.1*

NOTE: Bold line is average percentage reclaimed water by year, light lines are the percentage reclaimed water for individual service areas in ZIP.

Figure C.1—Percentage of Reclaimed Water for ZIP Codes in the Montebello Forebay Region: Weighted Average and Individual Service Areas

Table C.2

Estimated Annual Percentage of Reclaimed Water for Montebello Forebay Water System Service Areas, 1981–1995

Map No.	Water System	1981	1982	1983	1984	1985	1986	1987	1988	1989	1990	1991	1992	1993	1994	1995
1A	CAWATER	0	0	0	0	0	0	0	0	0	0	0	0	0	0	0
1B	CAWATER	1	1	2	1	2	3	3	3	2	3	4	1	1	2	2
1C	CAWATER	1	0	1	1	1	1	1	2	1	2	6	0	1	4	2
1D	CAWATER	0	0	0	0	0	0	0	0	0	0	0	0	0	0	0
1E	CAWATER	5	1	3	2	5	6	3	6	5	6	10	1	4	4	6
3A	DOWNEY	17	15	14	19	14	19	18	21	24	27	29	28	28	28	22
3B	DOWNEY	18	20	10	15	14	10	13	15	13	25	27	23	21	32	24
3C	DOWNEY	20	18	15	13	17	18	12	20	17	19	23	21	26	30	32
3D	DOWNEY	9	14	15	19	21	9	21	20	17	25	30	29	31	33	22
3E	DOWNEY	8	11	9	14	14	15	15	11	18	20	20	20	23	24	19
3F	DOWNEY	20	10	14	12	16	17		18	16	16	25	30	28	31	33
5	COMMERCE	0	0	0	0	0	0	0	0	0	0	0	0	0	0	0
6	LAHAB	19	5	6	20	14	13	21	21	18	27	25	11	6	23	9
7	MUTUAL	19	21	9	21	20	17	25	30	29	31	33	22	20	38	16
8A	MONTCITY	19	0	0	0	0	0	0	0	0	0	0	0	0	0	0
8B	MONTCITY	0	0	0	0	0	0	0	0	0	0	0	0	0	0	0
8C	MONTCITY	19	21	5	14	19	16	21	27	17	25	30	22	12	17	7
9	MONTL&W	14	14	18	20	9	20	15	16	23	28	27	29	31	21	19
10A	NORWALK	15	19	14	21	20	17	25	30	29	31	21	18	11	15	13
10B	NORWALK	11	15	11	16	12	10	9	17	16	15	13	5	4	21	7
10C	NORWALK	12	16	16	7	12	13	12	20	17	20	20	17	25	30	29
10D	NORWALK	0	0	0	0	0	0	0	0	0	0	0	0	0	0	0
10E	NORWALK	0	0	0	0	0	0	0	0	0	0	0	0	0	0	0
10F	NORWALK	0	0	0	0	0	7	10	11	13	12	10	4	2	17	5

Table C.2—continued

Map No.	Water System	1981	1982	1983	1984	1985	1986	1987	1988	1989	1990	1991	1992	1993	1994	1995
11A	ORCHARD	14	6	4	13	10	7	12	17	10	17	20	12	10	21	8
11B	ORCHARD	14	6	4	13	10	7	12	17	10	17	20	12	10	21	8
12A	PARK	0	0	0	0	0	0	0	0	0	0	0	0	0	0	0
12B	PARK	1	19	21	9	12	8	11	14	13	20	16	17	22	27	28
12C	PARK	1	19	21	9	12	8	11	14	13	20	16	17	22	27	28
12D	PARK	1	19	21	9	12	8	11	14	13	20	16	17	22	27	28
12E	PARK	1	1	1	1	1	1	2	1	3	3	2	1	2	1	4
12F	PARK	0	0	0	0	0	0	0	0	0	0	0	0	0	0	0
12G	PARK	1	1	1	1	1	2	1	2	1	3	2	5	2	2	1
12H	PARK	13	15	14	8	1	1	1	1	2	3	20	13	6	4	5
12I	PARK	10	6	3	5	8	12	12	5	9	7	11	13	4	4	3
12J	PARK	0	0	0	0	0	0	0	0	1	1	1	1	1	0	0
13	PICO	16	17	17	17	18	20	21	19	28	29	25	28	28	19	24
14A	PICORIV	19	20	9	21	20	17	25	30	29	31	33	22	20	38	16
14B	PICORIV	16	17	13	21	13	20	22	21	26	30	31	27	27	33	17
14C	PICORIV	9	8	6	12	7	8	13	14	10	23	12	11	8	21	16
14D	PICORIV	0	0	0	0	0	0	0	0	0	0	0	0	0	0	0
15A	SANGAB	0	0	0	0	0	0	0	0	0	0	0	0	0	0	0
15B	SANGAB	0	0	0	0	0	0	0	0	0	0	0	0	0	0	0
15C	SANGAB	0	0	0	0	0	0	0	0	0	0	0	0	0	0	0
15D	SANGAB	21	12	18	20	17	23	29	29	30	33	26	21	28	25	25
15E	SANGAB	0	0	0	0	0	0	0	0	0	0	0	0	0	0	0
16A	SFS	11	15	11	16	12	10	14	17	16	15	16	7	6	25	9
16B	SFS	NA	NA	NA	NA	NA	NA	NA	NA	NA	NA	NA	NA	NA	NA	NA
16C	SFS	NA	NA	NA	NA	NA	NA	NA	NA	NA	NA	NA	NA	NA	NA	NA
17	S MONTEB	19	21	9	21	20	17	25	30	29	31	33	22	24	37	16

Table C.2—continued

Map No.	Water System	1981	1982	1983	1984	1985	1986	1987	1988	1989	1990	1991	1992	1993	1994	1995
18A	S CA WATER	7	8	8	3	6	5	6	12	8	13	16	26	10	22	18
18B	S CA WATER	8	5	8	6	9	8	4	14	10	11	15	27	9	25	24
18C	S CA WATER	7	11	7	4	4	7	9	11	7	11	10	11	11	15	13
18D	S CA WATER	0	1	0	0	0	0	0	0	0	0	0	0	0	0	0
18E	S CA WATER	13	10	13	13	19	16	10	15	13	18	19	10	15	15	17
18F	S CA WATER	17	14	15	17	23	21	9	14	15	19	21	9	21	20	17
18G	S CA WATER	18	20	10	15	14	10	13	15	13	25	27	23	21	32	24
18H	S CA WATER	0	0	0	0	0	0	0	0	0	0	0	0	0	0	0
19A	SUBURB	0	0	0	0	0	0	0	0	0	0	0	0	0	0	0
19B	SUBURB	0	0	0	0	0	0	0	0	0	0	0	1	1	0	0
19C	SUBURB	0	0	0	0	0	0	0	0	0	0	0	0	0	0	0
20	WHITTIER	0	0	0	0	0	0	0	0	0	0	0	0	0	0	0
24A	LYNWOOD	1	1	0	0	1	0	0	0	1	3	5	2	3	2	1
24B	LYNWOOD	1	2	3	4	4	6	7	7	5	5	6	4	3	3	1
25	MAYWOOD #3	0	0	0	0	0	0	0	0	0	0	0	0	0	0	0
26A	PEERLESS	17	23	15	15	17	23	21	9	14	15	19	21	9	21	20
26B	PEERLESS	17	23	15	15	17	23	21	9	14	15	19	21	9	21	20
26C	PEERLESS	17	23	20	5	4	2	0	0	0	0	1	0	0	0	0
26D	PEERLESS	2	2	3	7	6	6	12	11	11	7	5	8	14	14	7
26E	PEERLESS	0	0	0	0	0	0	0	0	0	0	0	0	0	0	0
26F	PEERLESS	0	0	0	0	0	0	0	0	0	0	0	0	0	0	0
26G	PEERLESS	0	0	0	0	0	0	0	0	0	0	0	0	0	0	0
28	RANCHOLOS	12	15	11	8	13	14	14	16	14	14	11	14	9	8	13
30A	SOUTHGATE	1	1	10	7	9	8	11	14	13	20	16	17	22	27	28
30B	SOUTHGATE	1	19	21	9	12	8	11	14	13	20	16	17	22	27	28
31	TR180	0	0	0	0	0	0	0	0	0	0	0	0	0	0	0

Table C.2—continued

Map No.	Water System	1981	1982	1983	1984	1985	1986	1987	1988	1989	1990	1991	1992	1993	1994	1995
32	TR349	0	0	0	0	0	0	0	0	0	0	0	0	0	0	0
33A	BELFLWR-SOM	2	2	6	4	5	3	5	4	1	2	2	3	4	2	6
33B	BELFLWR-SOM	5	6	5	2	3	4	5	4	1	2	2	3	4	2	6
34	HUN	0	0	0	0	0	0	0	0	0	0	0	0	0	0	0
35	PARAM	1	2	1	2	2	3	4	6	3	3	4	2	2	1	2
36	BHG	0	0	0	0	0	0	0	0	0	0	0	0	0	0	0
37	BIGBY	0	0	0	0	0	0	0	0	0	0	0	0	0	0	0
39A	COUNTY	2	2	6	4	5	3	5	4	1	2	2	3	4	2	6
39B	COUNTY	0	0	0	0	0	0	0	0	0	0	0	0	0	0	0
43	MAYWOOD #1	0	0	0	0	0	0	0	0	0	0	0	0	0	0	0
44	MAYWOOD #2	0	0	0	0	0	0	0	0	0	0	0	0	0	0	0
46	WALNUT PARK	0	0	0	0	0	0	0	0	0	0	0	0	0	0	0
47	BEVERLY ACRES	0	0	0	0	0	0	0	0	0	0	0	0	0	0	0
48	INDUSTRY	0	0	0	0	0	0	0	0	0	0	0	0	0	0	0
49	LADWP	0	0	0	0	0	0	0	0	0	0	0	0	0	0	0
50	VERNON	0	0	0	0	0	0	0	0	0	0	0	0	0	0	0

Table C.3

Estimated Annual Percentage of Reclaimed Water for ZIP Codes in Montebello Forebay Region, 1981–1993

ZIP Code	1981	1982	1983	1984	1985	1986	1987	1988	1989	1990	1991	1992	1993
90022	0.46	0.15	0.61	0.46	0.61	0.77	0.77	1.07	0.61	1.07	2.43	0.08	0.46
90023	0.02	0.01	0.04	0.02	0.04	0.05	0.05	0.06	0.04	0.06	0.11	0.01	0.02
90040	1.55	0.65	1.12	1.40	1.55	1.46	1.62	2.77	1.49	2.71	6.74	0.68	1.34
90063	0.22	0.22	0.43	0.22	0.43	0.65	0.65	0.65	0.43	0.65	0.87	0.11	0.22
90201	5.37	4.96	5.69	4.11	6.52	5.47	4.33	7.44	5.69	8.49	9.68	10.65	6.81
90240	12.92	13.10	12.05	16.69	14.58	16.59	16.97	16.77	20.74	23.57	25.27	24.92	26.20
90241	18.35	17.32	12.49	13.74	15.49	14.53	13.23	17.15	15.38	21.06	24.59	22.79	24.06
90242	17.70	19.75	10.05	14.65	13.95	10.20	13.05	15.05	13.05	24.45	26.20	22.55	20.40
90255	0.00	0.00	0.00	0.00	0.00	0.00	0.00	0.00	0.00	0.00	0.00	0.00	0.00
90262	0.73	1.45	1.69	2.25	2.41	3.38	3.94	3.94	3.19	3.84	5.06	2.96	2.78
90270	0.00	0.00	0.00	0.00	0.00	0.00	0.00	0.00	0.00	0.00	0.00	0.00	0.00
90280	1.56	2.01	10.49	7.39	9.56	8.44	10.90	13.96	13.03	19.91	16.13	16.67	21.90
90601	0.00	0.00	0.00	0.00	0.00	0.00	0.00	0.00	0.00	0.00	0.00	0.00	0.00
90602	0.00	0.00	0.00	0.00	0.00	0.00	0.00	0.00	0.00	0.00	0.00	0.01	0.01
90603	0.00	0.00	0.00	0.00	0.00	0.00	0.00	0.00	0.00	0.00	0.00	0.11	0.11
90604	5.47	2.34	1.56	5.08	3.91	2.73	4.69	6.64	3.91	6.64	7.81	4.69	3.91
90605	1.02	0.65	0.29	0.95	0.73	0.51	0.87	1.24	0.73	1.24	1.46	0.89	0.74
90606	16.28	9.43	13.87	15.54	13.24	17.79	22.47	22.53	23.28	25.60	20.27	16.32	21.65
90631	18.93	4.98	5.98	19.92	13.95	12.95	20.92	20.92	17.93	26.89	24.90	10.96	5.98
90640	10.56	10.84	8.32	12.41	9.02	11.62	12.23	14.22	15.60	18.16	18.80	15.88	16.59
90650	6.10	6.99	5.11	3.74	3.53	5.22	5.61	5.53	5.04	6.35	8.73	8.75	5.87
90660	14.40	14.76	11.55	16.47	14.62	15.52	19.34	19.85	22.34	27.55	22.89	21.22	19.84
90670	13.34	14.20	12.62	16.88	13.14	13.08	17.53	19.80	19.28	19.25	18.32	10.35	11.26
90706	2.93	3.39	4.36	2.74	3.40	3.08	4.41	3.28	1.86	2.42	2.24	2.78	3.58
90723	1.67	2.49	1.58	2.62	2.87	3.73	4.17	6.28	3.48	3.65	4.68	2.28	2.79

MINIMUM DETECTABLE ODDS RATIO FOR EACH
OUTCOME AND EXPOSURE GROUP

Table D.1

Minimum Detectable Odds Ratio by Outcome and Exposure Group

Outcome	Exposure Group	Minimum Odds Ratio
Low birth weight (all gestational ages)	More than 0 to <2% (RW 1)	1.07
	2–<5% (RW 2)	1.07
	5–<15% (RW 3)	1.06
	15% or higher (RW 4)	1.08
Low birth weight (full-term births only)	More than 0 to <2% (RW 1)	1.09
	2–<5% (RW 2)	1.10
	5–<15% (RW 3)	1.09
	15% or higher (RW 4)	1.12
Very low birth weight (all gestational ages)	More than 0 to <2% (RW 1)	1.16
	2–<5% (RW 2)	1.17
	5–<15% (RW 3)	1.15
	15% or higher (RW 4)	1.20
Preterm birth	More than 0 to <2% (RW 1)	1.07
	2–<5% (RW 2)	1.08
	5–<15% (RW 3)	1.06
	15% or higher (RW 4)	1.09
Infant mortality	More than 0 to <2% (RW 1)	1.18
	2–<5% (RW 2)	1.20
	5–<15% (RW 3)	1.17
	15% or higher (RW 4)	1.23
Chromosomal syndromes	More than 0 to <2% (RW 1)	1.60
	2–<5% (RW 2)	1.64
	5–<15% (RW 3)	1.56
	15% or higher (RW 4)	1.54
Syndromes other than chromosomal	More than 0 to <2% (RW 1)	1.95
	2–<5% (RW 2)	2.03
	5–<15% (RW 3)	1.89
	15% or higher (RW 4)	1.85

Table D.1—continued

Outcome	Exposure Group	Minimum Odds Ratio
All defects	More than 0 to <2% (RW 1)	1.20
	2–<5% (RW 2)	1.22
	5–<15% (RW 3)	1.19
	15% or higher (RW 4)	1.19
Neural tube defects	More than 0 to <2% (RW 1)	3.17
	2–<5% (RW 2)	3.38
	5–<15% (RW 3)	3.00
	15% or higher (RW 4)	2.88
Other nervous system defects	More than 0 to <2% (RW 1)	1.62
	2–<5% (RW 2)	1.67
	5–<15% (RW 3)	1.59
	15% or higher (RW 4)	1.56
Ears, eyes, face, and neck defects	More than 0 to <2% (RW 1)	1.42
	2–<5% (RW 2)	1.44
	5–<15% (RW 3)	1.39
	15% or higher (RW 4)	1.38
Major cardiac defects	More than 0 to <2% (RW 1)	1.49
	2–<5% (RW 2)	1.52
	5–<15% (RW 3)	1.46
	15% or higher (RW 4)	1.44
Patent ductus arteriosus	More than 0 to <2% (RW 1)	1.94
	2–<5% (RW 2)	2.01
	5–<15% (RW 3)	1.88
	15% or higher (RW 4)	1.84
Other heart defects	More than 0 to <2% (RW 1)	1.70
	2–<5% (RW 2)	1.75
	5–<15% (RW 3)	1.66
	15% or higher (RW 4)	1.63
Respiratory system defects	More than 0 to <2% (RW 1)	1.64
	2–<5% (RW 2)	1.68
	5–<15% (RW 3)	1.60
	15% or higher (RW 4)	1.57
Cleft defects	More than 0 to <2% (RW 1)	1.96
	2–<5% (RW 2)	2.03
	5–<15% (RW 3)	1.90
	15% or higher (RW 4)	1.85
Pyloric stenosis	More than 0 to <2% (RW 1)	1.74
	2–<5% (RW 2)	1.80
	5–<15% (RW 3)	1.70
	15% or higher (RW 4)	1.66
Intestinal atresias	More than 0 to <2% (RW 1)	2.14
	2–<5% (RW 2)	2.23
	5–<15% (RW 3)	2.06
	15% or higher (RW 4)	2.01

Table D.1—continued

Outcome	Exposure Group	Minimum Odds Ratio
Other digestive system defects	More than 0 to <2% (RW 1)	1.60
	2–<5% (RW 2)	1.64
	5–<15% (RW 3)	1.56
	15% or higher (RW 4)	1.54
Urogenital system defects	More than 0 to <2% (RW 1)	1.50
	2–<5% (RW 2)	1.53
	5–<15% (RW 3)	1.47
	15% or higher (RW 4)	1.45
Limb defects	More than 0 to <2% (RW 1)	3.19
	2–<5% (RW 2)	3.40
	5–<15% (RW 3)	3.02
	15% or higher (RW 4)	2.90
Other musculoskeletal defects	More than 0 to <2% (RW 1)	1.36
	2–<5% (RW 2)	1.39
	5–<15% (RW 3)	1.34
	15% or higher (RW 4)	1.33
Integument defects	More than 0 to <2% (RW 1)	1.60
	2–<5% (RW 2)	1.65
	5–<15% (RW 3)	1.57
	15% or higher (RW 4)	1.54
All other defects	More than 0 to <2% (RW 1)	3.03
	2–<5% (RW 2)	3.22
	5–<15% (RW 3)	2.88
	15% or higher (RW 4)	2.77

RESULTS OF SENSITIVITY ANALYSES USING LOGISTIC REGRESSION MODELS OF PRENATAL DEVELOPMENT OUTCOMES AND INFANT MORTALITY

Below is the key to the terminology used in Tables E.1 through E.5.

Characteristic	Variable in Model	Category
Mother's race/ethnicity	BLACK	African-American
	WHITE	Non-Hispanic White
	ASIAN	Asian
	RACEOTH	All other
	Reference category	Hispanic
Child's gender	MALE	Male child
	Reference category	Female child
Mother's age	L_M_AGEI	21–30 years
	M_M_AGEI	31 years and older
	VRYNGMOM	Less than 17 years
	Reference category	17–20 years
	BLKXLAII	Interaction term: BLACK and L_M_AGEI
	BLKXMAII	Interaction term: BLACK and M_M_AGEI
	BLKXVYMI	Interaction term: BLACK and VRYNGMOM
Birth order	FIRSTCHD	First child
	Reference category	Second child or later
Total number of children	TOTCHD4	Number (>3) of children born to mother
Median home value	LHOMEVAL	Log of median home value in dollars by ZIP code from 1990 census
Maternal medical problem on birth certificate	Cardiac disease	Diagnosis of cardiac disease
	Renal disease	Diagnosis of renal disease
	Reference category	Neither diagnosis
Birthplace of mother	BPLMMX	Mexico
	BPLMUS	United States
	Reference category	Another country
Number of infants born to mother who died	NLBIRDIE	Count of previous infants who died
Interval since last live birth	BIRTHINT	Number of months since last live birth (for non-first-born children)
Month prenatal care began	MNPRECRN	Coded 1–9 for month of pregnancy, 10 if no prenatal care
Gestational age	GA-37	Number of weeks of gestation minus 37
Residence in ZIP code receiving reclaimed water	EXPLOW	More than 0 to <2%
	EXPMED	2–<5%
	EXPHI	5–<15%
	EXPVHI	15% or higher

103

Table E.1

Adjusted Odds Ratios and 95 Percent Confidence Intervals for Low Birth Weight Among Full-Term Births for All Variables in Four Logistic Regression Models

| | Model 1 (N = 330,438) | | | Model 2 (N = 301,890) | | | Model 3 (N = 333,161) | | | Model 4 (N = 304,501) | | |
| | | 95% CI | | | 95% CI | | | 95% CI | | | 95% CI | |
	OR	Lower	Upper	OR	Lower	Upper	OR	Lower	Upper	OR	Lower	Upper
Intercept	0.85	0.18	4.08	0.62	0.06	6.16	0.03	0.03	0.04	0.03	0.03	0.04
BLACK	1.51	1.26	1.83	1.41	1.24	1.59	1.81	1.51	2.18	1.68	1.49	1.90
WHITE	1.07	0.99	1.15	1.07	0.98	1.17	1.13	1.05	1.22	1.14	1.04	1.23
ASIAN	1.21	1.07	1.35	1.20	1.05	1.36	1.35	1.18	1.55	1.36	1.18	1.57
RACEOTH	1.16	1.00	1.34	1.15	0.98	1.33	1.42	1.25	1.61	1.43	1.24	1.64
MALE	0.73	0.70	0.76	0.73	0.70	0.76	0.77	0.74	0.81	0.77	0.74	0.81
L_M_AGEI	0.97	0.88	1.08	0.97	0.87	1.09	0.80	0.74	0.86	0.80	0.73	0.86
M_M_AGEI	0.96	0.89	1.03	0.96	0.88	1.04	0.76	0.71	0.81	0.76	0.71	0.81
VRYNGMOM	1.03	0.89	1.19	0.99	0.85	1.15	1.28	1.12	1.46	1.23	1.07	1.41
BLKXLAII	1.38	1.09	1.76	1.47	1.22	1.77	1.50	1.18	1.91	1.58	1.31	1.91
BLKXMAII	1.34	1.09	1.64	1.37	1.20	1.57	1.40	1.17	1.69	1.42	1.25	1.61
BLKXVYMI	0.85	0.53	1.35	0.83	0.36	1.89	0.86	0.54	1.38	0.81	0.36	1.83
FIRSTCHD	2.00	1.85	2.15	2.04	1.88	2.21						
TOTCHLD4	1.01	1.00	1.03	1.01	0.99	1.03						
LHOMEVAL	0.80	0.70	0.91	0.82	0.68	0.99						
cardiac disease	2.43	1.80	3.28	2.63	1.95	3.55						
renal disease	1.53	0.65	3.62	1.81	0.80	4.12						
BPLMMX	0.84	0.77	0.91	0.83	0.76	0.91						
BPLMUS	1.04	0.96	1.11	1.02	0.95	1.09						
NLBIRDIE	1.16	1.04	1.29	1.18	1.06	1.32						
BIRTHINT	1.00	1.00	1.00	1.00	1.00	1.00						
MNPRECRN	1.07	1.06	1.09	1.07	1.06	1.08						
GA-37	0.56	0.54	0.57	0.56	0.54	0.57						
EXPLOW	0.98	0.90	1.06	1.00	0.91	1.09	1.00	0.93	1.09	1.02	0.94	1.11

Table E.1—continued

	Model 1 (N = 330,438)			Model 2 (N = 301,890)			Model 3 (N = 333,161)			Model 4 (N = 304,501)		
		95% CI			95% CI			95% CI			95% CI	
	OR	Lower	Upper	OR	Lower	Upper	OR	Lower	Upper	OR	Lower	Upper
EXPMED	0.95	0.89	1.01	0.97	0.90	1.04	0.97	0.91	1.02	0.99	0.93	1.05
EXPHI	0.96	0.90	1.02	0.97	0.91	1.03	0.97	0.91	1.02	0.98	0.93	1.04
EXPVHI	0.88	0.81	0.96	0.89	0.81	0.96	0.89	0.82	0.96	0.90	0.83	0.98

Model 1 = Full set of covariates with control area defined as San Fernando Valley and Pomona. Results reported in Chapter Four.

Model 2 = Full set of covariates with control area defined as San Fernando Valley only.

Model 3 = Limited set of covariates with control area defined as San Fernando Valley and Pomona.

Model 4 = Limited set of covariates with control area defined as San Fernando Valley only.

Table E.2

Adjusted Odds Ratios and 95 Percent Confidence Intervals for Low Birth Weight Among All Births for All Variables in Four Logistic Regression Models

| | Model 1 (N = 447,028) | | | Model 2 (N = 409,089) | | | Model 3 (N = 450,825) | | | Model 4 (N = 412,725) | | |
| | | 95% CI | | | 95% CI | | | 95% CI | | | 95% CI | |
	OR	Lower	Upper	OR	Lower	Upper	OR	Lower	Upper	OR	Lower	Upper
Intercept	0.54	0.15	1.96	0.78	0.10	5.87	0.05	0.05	0.06	0.05	0.05	0.06
BLACK	1.37	1.10	1.71	1.42	1.20	1.69	1.82	1.53	2.16	1.86	1.56	2.22
WHITE	1.08	1.02	1.14	1.10	1.03	1.17	1.09	1.02	1.16	1.09	1.02	1.18
ASIAN	1.16	1.06	1.27	1.17	1.05	1.29	1.15	1.02	1.29	1.14	1.01	1.28
RACEOTH	1.16	1.05	1.29	1.17	1.04	1.30	1.32	1.21	1.43	1.32	1.22	1.44
MALE	0.82	0.80	0.84	0.82	0.80	0.85	0.92	0.90	0.94	0.93	0.90	0.95
L_M_AGEI	1.12	1.05	1.20	1.13	1.05	1.22	0.93	0.88	0.99	0.94	0.89	1.01
M_M_AGEI	1.01	0.96	1.06	1.01	0.96	1.07	0.78	0.75	0.81	0.78	0.75	0.82
VRYNGMOM	0.99	0.89	1.11	0.97	0.86	1.09	1.31	1.19	1.43	1.28	1.16	1.41
BLKXLAII	1.36	1.05	1.76	1.36	1.10	1.69	1.58	1.27	1.96	1.57	1.31	1.88
BLKXMAII	1.36	1.07	1.74	1.30	1.07	1.59	1.54	1.31	1.80	1.52	1.29	1.78
BLKXVYMI	0.71	0.41	1.25	0.53	0.27	1.04	0.98	0.65	1.50	0.81	0.51	1.29
FIRSTCHD	1.88	1.80	1.97	1.91	1.82	2.00						
TOTCHLD4	1.01	0.99	1.02	1.01	0.99	1.02						
Cardiac disease	2.73	2.25	3.31	2.87	2.36	3.49						
Renal disease	2.69	1.53	4.72	3.04	1.74	5.32						
BPLMMX	0.89	0.84	0.94	0.88	0.83	0.93						
BPLMUS	1.10	1.05	1.16	1.09	1.05	1.14						
LHOMEVAL	0.83	0.74	0.92	0.80	0.68	0.95						
NLBIRDIE	1.26	1.19	1.32	1.25	1.18	1.32						
BIRTHINT	1.00	1.00	1.00	1.00	1.00	1.00						
MNPRECRN	1.02	1.01	1.03	1.02	1.01	1.03						
GA-37	0.65	0.65	0.66	0.65	0.64	0.66						
EXPLOW	0.97	0.91	1.04	0.97	0.89	1.05	1.00	0.96	1.05	1.01	0.96	1.06

Table E.2—continued

| | Model 1 (N = 447,028) | | | Model 2 (N = 409,089) | | | Model 3 (N = 450,825) | | | Model 4 (N = 412,725) | | |
| | | 95% CI | | | 95% CI | | | 95% CI | | | 95% CI | |
	OR	Lower	Upper	OR	Lower	Upper	OR	Lower	Upper	OR	Lower	Upper
EXPMED	0.92	0.88	0.96	0.91	0.86	0.97	0.97	0.93	1.00	0.97	0.93	1.01
EXPHI	0.93	0.88	0.98	0.93	0.87	0.98	0.96	0.92	1.00	0.97	0.92	1.02
EXPVHI	0.91	0.84	0.98	0.91	0.84	0.99	0.95	0.88	1.03	0.96	0.88	1.04

Model 1 = Full set of covariates with control area defined as San Fernando Valley and Pomona.. Results reported in Chapter Four.
Model 2 = Full set of covariates with control area defined as San Fernando Valley only.
Model 3 = Limited set of covariates with control area defined as San Fernando Valley and Pomona.
Model 4 = Limited set of covariates with control area defined as San Fernando Valley only.

Table E.3
Adjusted Odds Ratios and 95 Percent Confidence Intervals for Very Low Birth Weight Among All Births for All Variables in Four Logistic Regression Models

| | Model 1 (N = 447,028) | | | Model 2 (N = 409,089) | | | Model 3 (N = 450,825) | | | Model 4 (N = 412,725) | | |
| | | 95% CI | | | 95% CI | | | 95% CI | | | 95% CI | |
	OR	Lower	Upper	OR	Lower	Upper	OR	Lower	Upper	OR	Lower	Upper
Intercept	0.13	0.01	2.58	0.03	0.00	2.37	0.01	0.01	0.01	0.01	0.01	0.01
BLACK	1.30	0.74	2.28	1.43	0.67	3.05	1.95	1.30	2.92	2.17	1.33	3.55
WHITE	0.88	0.77	1.00	0.88	0.76	1.02	0.88	0.79	0.98	0.89	0.79	1.00
ASIAN	0.85	0.62	1.16	0.76	0.53	1.08	0.71	0.52	0.97	0.64	0.48	0.85
RACEOTH	0.91	0.67	1.24	0.93	0.67	1.29	0.98	0.79	1.21	1.00	0.81	1.23
MALE	0.93	0.86	1.00	0.92	0.85	1.00	1.04	0.99	1.10	1.04	0.99	1.10
L_M_AGEI	1.52	1.21	1.91	1.55	1.21	1.98	1.17	1.04	1.31	1.20	1.06	1.36
M_M_AGEI	1.15	0.99	1.35	1.20	1.02	1.40	0.84	0.75	0.94	0.86	0.77	0.97
VRYNGMOM	0.85	0.64	1.12	0.90	0.67	1.20	1.16	0.90	1.50	1.17	0.89	1.54
BLKXLAII	1.03	0.57	1.86	1.12	0.49	2.58	1.66	1.10	2.51	1.56	0.98	2.50
BLKXMAII	1.29	0.75	2.22	1.21	0.57	2.58	1.70	1.19	2.44	1.62	1.02	2.59
BLKXVYMI	0.35	0.13	0.92	0.33	0.07	1.47	1.03	0.61	1.74	1.05	0.57	1.95
FIRSTCHD	1.85	1.66	2.07	1.81	1.60	2.03						
TOTCHLD4	0.99	0.95	1.03	0.99	0.95	1.04						
LMEDVAL	0.74	0.58	0.95	0.83	0.58	1.17						
cardiac disease	4.08	2.99	5.57	4.22	3.04	5.85						
renal disease	2.60	0.94	7.23	3.05	1.10	8.46						
BPLMMX	1.01	0.87	1.17	1.01	0.87	1.18						
BPLMUS	1.04	0.90	1.21	1.05	0.91	1.22						
NLBIRDIE	1.39	1.17	1.65	1.33	1.10	1.61						
BIRTHINT	1.00	1.00	1.01	1.00	1.00	1.01						
MNPRECRN	0.93	0.90	0.95	0.93	0.91	0.96						
GA-37	0.58	0.57	0.59	0.58	0.57	0.59						
EXPLOW	0.85	0.75	0.96	0.89	0.75	1.05	0.95	0.86	1.06	0.97	0.87	1.08

Table E.3—continued

| | Model 1 (N = 447,028) | | | Model 2 (N =409,089) | | | Model 3 (N = 450,825) | | | Model 4 (N = 412,725) | | |
| | | 95% CI | | | 95% CI | | | 95% CI | | | 95% CI | |
	OR	Lower	Upper	OR	Lower	Upper	OR	Lower	Upper	OR	Lower	Upper
EXPMED	0.90	0.76	1.07	0.92	0.74	1.14	0.98	0.91	1.07	0.99	0.90	1.09
EXPHI	1.07	0.92	1.24	1.10	0.93	1.29	1.05	0.95	1.17	1.07	0.96	1.19
EXPVHI	1.00	0.89	1.13	1.03	0.90	1.17	1.03	0.92	1.16	1.05	0.93	1.19

Model 1 = Full set of covariates with control area defined as San Fernando Valley and Pomona. Results reported in Chapter Four.

Model 2 = Full set of covariates with control area defined as San Fernando Valley only.

Model 3 = Limited set of covariates with control area defined as San Fernando Valley and Pomona.

Model 4 = Limited set of covariates with control area defined as San Fernando Valley only.

Table E.4

Adjusted Odds Ratios and 95 Percent Confidence Intervals for Preterm Births for All Variables in Four Logistic Regression Models

	Model 1 (N = 447,248)			Model 2 (N = 409,289)			Model 3 (N = 451,051)			Model 4 (N = 412,931)		
		95% CI			95% CI			95% CI			95% CI	
	OR	Lower	Upper	OR	Lower	Upper	OR	Lower	Upper	OR	Lower	Upper
Intercept	0.22	0.04	1.13	1.38	0.23	8.30	0.09	0.09	0.10	0.09	0.09	0.10
BLACK	1.30	1.13	1.49	1.28	1.08	1.53	1.44	1.25	1.66	1.42	1.17	1.72
WHITE	0.79	0.75	0.83	0.79	0.75	0.84	0.82	0.78	0.87	0.83	0.78	0.88
ASIAN	0.91	0.80	1.04	0.90	0.79	1.04	0.93	0.80	1.08	0.90	0.77	1.05
RACEOTH	1.03	0.97	1.08	1.03	0.97	1.09	1.07	1.01	1.14	1.07	1.00	1.14
MALE	1.13	1.10	1.16	1.14	1.10	1.17	1.13	1.10	1.16	1.14	1.11	1.17
L_M_AGEI	0.89	0.85	0.94	0.91	0.87	0.96	0.88	0.84	0.93	0.89	0.85	0.94
M_M_AGEI	0.80	0.77	0.82	0.80	0.78	0.83	0.77	0.75	0.79	0.77	0.75	0.79
VRYNGMOM	1.26	1.19	1.34	1.27	1.19	1.35	1.33	1.25	1.40	1.33	1.26	1.41
BLKX1AII	1.29	1.15	1.45	1.32	1.14	1.54	1.30	1.17	1.45	1.33	1.16	1.53
BLKXMAII	1.31	1.15	1.49	1.36	1.19	1.55	1.32	1.16	1.50	1.37	1.20	1.55
BLKXVYMI	1.28	1.01	1.62	1.34	0.94	1.91	1.28	1.00	1.62	1.32	0.93	1.89
FIRSTCHD	0.98	0.94	1.03	0.97	0.93	1.03						
TOTCHLD4	1.04	1.03	1.04	1.04	1.03	1.04						
LMEDVAL	0.92	0.80	1.05	0.79	0.68	0.91						
cardiac disease	2.15	1.82	2.54	2.15	1.81	2.57						
renal disease	2.53	1.69	3.79	2.64	1.72	4.05						
BPLMMX	0.85	0.82	0.88	0.84	0.81	0.87						
BPLMUS	1.04	1.00	1.08	1.05	1.00	1.10						
NLBIRDIE	1.17	1.10	1.24	1.16	1.09	1.23						
BIRTHINT	1.00	1.00	1.00	1.00	1.00	1.00						
MNPRECRN	1.08	1.07	1.09	1.08	1.07	1.09						
EXPLOW	0.98	0.93	1.04	0.93	0.88	0.98	1.00	0.95	1.05	0.99	0.95	1.04
EXPMED	1.03	0.95	1.11	0.98	0.92	1.04	1.04	0.96	1.12	1.03	0.96	1.11

Table E.4—continued

	Model 1 (N = 447,248)			Model 2 (N = 409,289)			Model 3 (N = 451,051)			Model 4 (N = 412,931)		
		95% CI			95% CI			95% CI			95% CI	
	OR	Lower	Upper	OR	Lower	Upper	OR	Lower	Upper	OR	Lower	Upper
EXPHI	1.02	0.97	1.06	0.98	0.94	1.02	1.03	0.99	1.07	1.02	0.98	1.06
EXPVHI	0.99	0.94	1.05	0.97	0.92	1.02	0.99	0.93	1.05	0.98	0.92	1.05

Model 1 = Full set of covariates with control area defined as San Fernando Valley and Pomona. Results reported in Chapter Four.

Model 2 = Full set of covariates with control area defined as San Fernando Valley only.

Model 3 = Limited set of covariates with control area defined as San Fernando Valley and Pomona.

Model 4 = Limited set of covariates with control area defined as San Fernando Valley only.

Table E.5
Adjusted Odds Ratios and 95 Percent Confidence Intervals for Infant Mortality for All Variables in Four Logistic Regression Models

| | Model 1 (N=460,866) | | | Model 2 (N=421,752) | | | Model 3 (N=465,258) | | | Model 4 (N=425,948) | | |
| | | 95% CI | | | 95% CI | | | 95% CI | | | 95% CI | |
	OR	Lower	Upper	OR	Lower	Upper	OR	Lower	Upper	OR	Lower	Upper
Intercept	0.03	0.00	0.79	0.06	0.00	6.01	0.01	0.01	0.01	0.01	0.01	0.01
BLACK	1.53	1.19	1.97	1.77	1.34	2.33	1.77	1.42	2.20	1.95	1.52	2.51
WHITE	1.14	1.00	1.30	1.16	1.01	1.34	1.21	1.08	1.36	1.22	1.08	1.38
ASIAN	1.00	0.72	1.39	1.01	0.69	1.47	0.89	0.64	1.24	0.92	0.64	1.32
RACEOTH	1.17	0.91	1.50	1.16	0.90	1.48	1.12	0.90	1.39	1.13	0.92	1.39
MALE	1.29	1.19	1.40	1.28	1.18	1.40	1.29	1.20	1.40	1.29	1.18	1.40
L_M_AGEI	0.91	0.79	1.06	0.97	0.85	1.12	0.88	0.78	0.99	0.92	0.82	1.03
M_M_AGEI	0.79	0.71	0.89	0.82	0.72	0.93	0.77	0.69	0.85	0.78	0.70	0.87
VRYNGMOM	1.21	0.96	1.52	1.24	0.98	1.58	1.26	1.01	1.58	1.29	1.01	1.63
BLKXLAII	1.36	0.88	2.11	1.26	0.74	2.14	1.29	0.85	1.97	1.23	0.73	2.07
BLKXMAII	1.33	1.00	1.77	1.23	0.86	1.75	1.31	0.98	1.75	1.24	0.88	1.75
BLKXVYMI	0.79	0.30	2.06	0.56	0.18	1.76	0.76	0.29	1.99	0.54	0.17	1.77
FIRSTCHD	0.92	0.82	1.03	0.93	0.83	1.05						
TOTCHLD4	1.02	1.00	1.05	1.02	0.99	1.04						
LHOMEVAL	0.86	0.66	1.11	0.81	0.56	1.18						
cardiac disease	2.47	1.63	3.73	2.48	1.58	3.89						
renal disease	3.10	1.26	7.60	3.55	1.50	8.40						
BPLMMX	1.05	0.90	1.23	1.04	0.88	1.22						
BPLMUS	1.26	1.08	1.47	1.21	1.03	1.42						
NLBIRDIE	1.51	1.35	1.68	1.52	1.35	1.71						
BIRTHINT	1.00	1.00	1.00	1.00	1.00	1.00						
MNPRECRN	1.06	1.04	1.08	1.06	1.03	1.08						
EXPLOW	1.05	0.92	1.21	1.04	0.87	1.24	1.10	0.99	1.23	1.13	1.00	1.27

Table E.5—continued

	Model 1 (N = 460,866)			Model 2 (N = 421,752)			Model 3 (N = 465,258)			Model 4 (N = 425,948)		
		95% CI			95% CI			95% CI			95% CI	
	OR	Lower	Upper	OR	Lower	Upper	OR	Lower	Upper	OR	Lower	Upper
EXPMED	1.05	0.92	1.19	1.03	0.87	1.22	1.09	0.98	1.22	1.11	0.98	1.25
EXPHI	1.04	0.90	1.19	1.03	0.89	1.20	1.05	0.92	1.21	1.08	0.94	1.23
EXPVHI	0.82	0.73	0.92	0.82	0.73	0.93	0.82	0.73	0.92	0.84	0.74	0.94

Model 1 = Full set of covariates with control area defined as San Fernando Valley and Pomona. Results reported in Chapter Four.
Model 2 = Full set of covariates with control area defined as San Fernando Valley only.
Model 3 = Limited set of covariates with control area defined as San Fernando Valley and Pomona.
Model 4 = Limited set of covariates with control area defined as San Fernando Valley only.

RESULTS OF SENSITIVITY ANALYSES USING LOGISTIC REGRESSION MODELS FOR BIRTH DEFECT OUTCOMES

Below is the key to the terminology used in Tables F.1 through F.19.

Characteristic	Variable in Model	Category
Birth year	B_YR90	Born in 1990
	B_YR91	Born in 1991
	B_YR93	Born in 1993
	Reference category	Born in 1992
Mother's race-ethnicity	BLACK	African-American
	WHITE	Non-Hispanic White
	ASIAN	Asian
	RACEOTH	All other
	Reference category	Hispanic
Mother's age	Y_M_AGEI	Less than 20 years
	L_M_AGEI	35 years and older
	Reference category	20–34 years
Child's gender	MALE	Male child
	Reference category	Female child
Mother's education	ELEMSCHL	Less than high school
	COLLPL	Some college or higher
	Reference category	High school
Adequacy of prenatal care	INADCAR2	Known to be inadequate (see definition in Table 3.5)
	Reference category	Unknown
Residence in ZIP code being served reclaimed water	EXPLOW	More than 0 to <2%
	EXPMED	2–<5%
	EXPHI	5–<15%
	EXPVHI	15% or higher

Table F.1
Adjusted Odds Ratios and 95 Percent Confidence Intervals for All Birth Defects for All Variables in Four Logistic Regression Models

Variable	Model 1 (N = 159,850)			Model 2 (N = 145,718)			Model 3 (N = 159,850)			Model 4 (N = 145,718)		
		95% CI			95% CI			95% CI			95% CI	
	OR	Lower	Upper	OR	Lower	Upper	OR	Lower	Upper	OR	Lower	Upper
INTERCEPT	0.01	0.01	0.01	0.01	0.01	0.02	0.01	0.01	0.01	0.01	0.01	0.02
B_YR90	1.17	1.02	1.35	1.17	1.01	1.36	1.17	1.02	1.35	1.17	1.01	1.36
B_YR91	0.99	0.89	1.11	1.00	0.89	1.12	1.00	0.89	1.11	1.00	0.89	1.12
B_YR93	0.89	0.80	1.00	0.90	0.80	1.01	0.89	0.80	0.99	0.90	0.80	1.01
BLACK	1.21	0.98	1.49	1.28	1.02	1.61	1.21	0.98	1.48	1.27	1.02	1.58
WHITE	1.28	1.17	1.41	1.27	1.15	1.41	1.27	1.17	1.39	1.25	1.15	1.37
ASIAN	1.05	0.76	1.46	1.04	0.72	1.52	1.04	0.75	1.44	1.02	0.71	1.48
RACEOTH	0.99	0.78	1.24	1.00	0.80	1.27	0.98	0.77	1.23	0.98	0.77	1.26
Y_M_AGE	1.00	0.88	1.15	1.02	0.89	1.17	1.01	0.89	1.14	1.03	0.91	1.17
L_M_AGE	1.00	0.87	1.16	1.01	0.87	1.18	1.00	0.86	1.16	1.01	0.86	1.18
MALE	1.50	1.37	1.64	1.52	1.39	1.67	1.50	1.37	1.64	1.52	1.39	1.66
ELEMSCHL	0.99	0.90	1.09	0.99	0.90	1.09						
COLLPL	0.98	0.86	1.12	0.96	0.84	1.09						
INADCAR2	1.07	0.90	1.29	1.10	0.91	1.32						
EXPLOW	0.98	0.87	1.11	0.92	0.84	1.00	0.98	0.88	1.11	0.92	0.84	1.00
EXPMED	1.04	0.87	1.23	0.96	0.82	1.13	1.04	0.87	1.23	0.97	0.83	1.13
EXPHI	0.94	0.83	1.06	0.88	0.79	0.97	0.94	0.83	1.06	0.88	0.80	0.97
EXPVHI	0.92	0.81	1.03	0.86	0.78	0.94	0.92	0.81	1.04	0.86	0.78	0.94

Model 1 = Full set of covariates with control area defined as San Fernando Valley and Pomona. Results reported in Chapter Four.
Model 2 = Full set of covariates with control area defined as San Fernando Valley only.
Model 3 = Limited set of covariates with control area defined as San Fernando Valley and Pomona.
Model 4 = Limited set of covariates with control area defined as San Fernando Valley only.

Table F.2

Adjusted Odds Ratios and 95 Percent Confidence Intervals for Neural Tube Defects for All Variables in Four Logistic Regression Models

Variable	Model 1 (N = 159,850)			Model 2 (N = 145,718)			Model 3 (N = 159,850)			Model 4 (N = 145,718)		
		95% CI			95% CI			95% CI			95% CI	
	OR	Lower	Upper	OR	Lower	Upper	OR	Lower	Upper	OR	Lower	Upper
INTERCEPT	0.00	0.00	0.00	0.00	0.00	0.00	0.00	0.00	0.00	0.00	0.00	0.00
B_YR90	1.77	1.01	3.10	1.95	1.10	3.46	1.78	1.02	3.11	1.96	1.11	3.47
B_YR91	0.99	0.54	1.82	0.99	0.52	1.91	1.00	0.54	1.82	0.99	0.52	1.91
B_YR93	0.77	0.38	1.53	0.79	0.38	1.67	0.76	0.38	1.51	0.79	0.37	1.65
BLACK	0.69	0.15	3.23	0.42	0.05	3.82	0.60	0.15	2.45	0.36	0.05	2.81
WHITE	0.40	0.14	1.14	0.43	0.15	1.24	0.34	0.13	0.89	0.36	0.14	0.95
ASIAN	0.65	0.08	5.12	0.76	0.09	6.03	0.58	0.07	4.79	0.65	0.08	5.46
RACEOTH	0.66	0.07	6.20	0.72	0.08	6.89	0.57	0.08	4.18	0.60	0.08	4.46
Y_M_AGE	1.11	0.57	2.17	0.96	0.47	1.94	1.08	0.56	2.09	0.94	0.48	1.88
L_M_AGE	0.56	0.20	1.61	0.43	0.13	1.45	0.60	0.21	1.71	0.46	0.14	1.53
MALE	1.07	0.65	1.76	0.99	0.59	1.66	1.07	0.65	1.76	0.99	0.59	1.66
ELEMSCHL	1.49	0.79	2.78	1.45	0.74	2.81						
COLLPL	0.99	0.46	2.12	0.92	0.41	2.07						
INADCAR2	1.02	0.44	2.35	1.10	0.47	2.56						
EXPLOW	1.52	1.03	2.24	1.47	0.97	2.23	1.51	1.02	2.24	1.47	0.97	2.24
EXPMED	1.44	0.90	2.29	1.43	0.88	2.32	1.43	0.88	2.33	1.43	0.86	2.37
EXPHI	1.55	0.96	2.50	1.52	0.92	2.49	1.52	0.95	2.41	1.49	0.92	2.41
EXPVHI	0.81	0.21	3.04	0.79	0.21	3.01	0.76	0.20	2.86	0.75	0.20	2.84

Model 1 = Full set of covariates with control area defined as San Fernando Valley and Pomona. Results reported in Chapter Four.
Model 2 = Full set of covariates with control area defined as San Fernando Valley only.
Model 3 = Limited set of covariates with control area defined as San Fernando Valley and Pomona.
Model 4 = Limited set of covariates with control area defined as San Fernando Valley only.

Table F.3

Adjusted Odds Ratios and 95 Percent Confidence Intervals for Other Nervous System Defects for All Variables in Four Logistic Regression Models

Variable	Model 1 (N = 159,850)			Model 2 (N = 145,718)			Model 3 (N = 159,850)			Model 4 (N = 145,718)		
		95% CI			95% CI			95% CI			95% CI	
	OR	Lower	Upper	OR	Lower	Upper	OR	Lower	Upper	OR	Lower	Upper
INTERCEPT	0.00	0.00	0.00	0.00	0.00	0.00	0.00	0.00	0.00	0.00	0.00	0.00
B_YR90	1.33	1.02	1.73	1.49	1.18	1.88	1.34	1.03	1.74	1.49	1.18	1.89
B_YR91	0.90	0.61	1.33	1.00	0.68	1.47	0.90	0.61	1.34	1.01	0.68	1.48
B_YR93	0.78	0.57	1.06	0.85	0.62	1.17	0.77	0.57	1.05	0.84	0.61	1.16
BLACK	1.83	1.02	3.27	2.19	1.21	3.98	1.60	0.90	2.84	1.87	1.02	3.42
WHITE	1.45	1.02	2.06	1.44	0.99	2.08	1.26	0.92	1.72	1.21	0.86	1.69
ASIAN	0.74	0.30	1.85	0.65	0.23	1.84	0.65	0.24	1.72	0.54	0.18	1.64
RACEOTH	1.32	0.70	2.50	1.45	0.77	2.72	1.11	0.61	2.03	1.16	0.63	2.12
Y_M_AGE	1.39	1.06	1.82	1.38	1.06	1.81	1.40	1.09	1.81	1.41	1.09	1.82
L_M_AGE	1.12	0.78	1.61	1.06	0.72	1.57	1.16	0.79	1.69	1.09	0.73	1.64
MALE	1.06	0.82	1.38	1.04	0.79	1.36	1.06	0.82	1.38	1.04	0.79	1.36
ELEMSCHL	1.34	0.99	1.80	1.35	1.01	1.81						
COLLPL	0.89	0.63	1.25	0.81	0.57	1.16						
INADCAR2	1.13	0.73	1.76	1.14	0.73	1.80						
EXPLOW	1.19	0.84	1.69	1.08	0.77	1.50	1.20	0.85	1.70	1.09	0.78	1.52
EXPMED	1.04	0.77	1.42	0.93	0.70	1.24	1.05	0.77	1.42	0.94	0.70	1.25
EXPHI	1.10	0.77	1.58	1.00	0.70	1.42	1.09	0.78	1.54	1.00	0.71	1.39
EXPVHI	0.89	0.66	1.19	0.81	0.61	1.08	0.86	0.63	1.16	0.78	0.58	1.05

Model 1 = Full set of covariates with control area defined as San Fernando Valley and Pomona. Results reported in Chapter Four.
Model 2 = Full set of covariates with control area defined as San Fernando Valley only.
Model 3 = Limited set of covariates with control area defined as San Fernando Valley and Pomona.
Model 4 = Limited set of covariates with control area defined as San Fernando Valley only.

Table F.4

Adjusted Odds Ratios and 95 Percent Confidence Intervals for Ears, Eyes, Face, and Neck Defects for All Variables in Four Logistic Regression Models

Variable	Model 1 (N = 159,850)			Model 2 (N = 145,718)			Model 3 (N = 159,850)			Model 4 (N = 145,718)		
		95% CI			95% CI			95% CI			95% CI	
	OR	Lower	Upper	OR	Lower	Upper	OR	Lower	Upper	OR	Lower	Upper
INTERCEPT	0.00	0.00	0.00	0.00	0.00	0.01	0.00	0.00	0.00	0.00	0.00	0.00
B_YR90	1.02	0.80	1.30	1.02	0.79	1.32	1.02	0.80	1.31	1.02	0.79	1.32
B_YR91	0.94	0.79	1.12	0.94	0.79	1.13	0.94	0.79	1.13	0.95	0.79	1.13
B_YR93	0.91	0.73	1.14	0.90	0.71	1.14	0.91	0.73	1.13	0.90	0.71	1.13
BLACK	0.59	0.38	0.93	0.69	0.44	1.08	0.54	0.36	0.82	0.62	0.40	0.94
WHITE	1.00	0.74	1.36	1.01	0.72	1.40	0.90	0.67	1.20	0.88	0.64	1.21
ASIAN	0.76	0.33	1.79	0.88	0.38	2.01	0.66	0.29	1.51	0.74	0.33	1.65
RACEOTH	1.56	1.02	2.39	1.57	1.00	2.46	1.30	0.81	2.08	1.27	0.78	2.07
Y_M_AGE	1.04	0.82	1.32	1.02	0.80	1.32	1.08	0.86	1.36	1.07	0.84	1.36
L_M_AGE	1.02	0.74	1.39	1.05	0.76	1.44	1.01	0.74	1.38	1.04	0.77	1.42
MALE	1.05	0.87	1.26	1.06	0.87	1.30	1.05	0.87	1.26	1.06	0.87	1.30
ELEMSCHL	1.05	0.87	1.27	1.09	0.90	1.31						
COLLPL	0.74	0.56	0.97	0.72	0.55	0.94						
INADCAR2	1.13	0.84	1.51	1.15	0.85	1.55						
EXPLOW	0.86	0.69	1.06	0.79	0.66	0.95	0.87	0.70	1.08	0.80	0.66	0.97
EXPMED	1.34	1.08	1.66	1.23	1.03	1.47	1.36	1.10	1.68	1.25	1.04	1.51
EXPHI	0.88	0.70	1.10	0.81	0.66	0.99	0.88	0.71	1.10	0.82	0.68	0.99
EXPVHI	0.89	0.73	1.09	0.82	0.69	0.99	0.88	0.71	1.08	0.81	0.68	0.97

Model 1 = Full set of covariates with control area defined as San Fernando Valley and Pomona. Results reported in Chapter Four.
Model 2 = Full set of covariates with control area defined as San Fernando Valley only.
Model 3 = Limited set of covariates with control area defined as San Fernando Valley and Pomona.
Model 4 = Limited set of covariates with control area defined as San Fernando Valley only.

Table F.5

Adjusted Odds Ratios and 95 Percent Confidence Intervals for Major Cardiac Defects for All Variables in Four Logistic Regression Models

Variable	Model 1 (N = 159,850)			Model 2 (N = 145,718)			Model 3 (N = 159,850)			Model 4 (N = 145,718)		
		95% CI			95% CI			95% CI			95% CI	
	OR	Lower	Upper	OR	Lower	Upper	OR	Lower	Upper	OR	Lower	Upper
INTERCEPT	0.00	0.00	0.00	0.00	0.00	0.00	0.00	0.00	0.00	0.00	0.00	0.00
B_YR90	1.16	0.85	1.60	1.19	0.84	1.68	1.17	0.85	1.61	1.20	0.84	1.70
B_YR91	0.84	0.65	1.08	0.92	0.72	1.18	0.85	0.66	1.09	0.93	0.72	1.19
B_YR93	0.87	0.66	1.15	0.91	0.68	1.23	0.86	0.65	1.14	0.91	0.67	1.22
BLACK	1.33	0.76	2.33	1.26	0.60	2.64	1.20	0.70	2.07	1.13	0.55	2.32
WHITE	1.57	1.14	2.17	1.58	1.12	2.23	1.41	1.08	1.84	1.40	1.06	1.84
ASIAN	1.16	0.50	2.66	1.36	0.61	3.03	1.06	0.47	2.38	1.21	0.55	2.67
RACEOTH	1.89	1.10	3.26	2.07	1.21	3.54	1.70	1.04	2.77	1.82	1.12	2.96
Y_M_AGE	1.08	0.82	1.42	1.12	0.84	1.48	1.08	0.82	1.40	1.12	0.85	1.48
L_M_AGE	1.05	0.71	1.56	1.09	0.73	1.63	1.08	0.73	1.61	1.12	0.75	1.68
MALE	1.23	1.05	1.45	1.28	1.09	1.50	1.23	1.05	1.45	1.28	1.09	1.50
ELEMSCHL	1.32	1.02	1.69	1.31	1.00	1.72						
COLLPL	0.99	0.77	1.27	0.95	0.74	1.23						
INADCAR2	1.28	0.89	1.84	1.30	0.89	1.89						
EXPLOW	1.17	1.01	1.35	1.15	0.98	1.34	1.18	1.02	1.36	1.16	0.99	1.35
EXPMED	0.92	0.72	1.17	0.90	0.70	1.15	0.92	0.72	1.17	0.91	0.71	1.16
EXPHI	1.14	0.92	1.42	1.12	0.88	1.42	1.13	0.90	1.42	1.11	0.87	1.42
EXPVHI	1.23	0.94	1.61	1.21	0.91	1.60	1.19	0.91	1.56	1.17	0.88	1.54

Model 1 = Full set of covariates with control area defined as San Fernando Valley and Pomona. Results reported in Chapter Four.

Model 2 = Full set of covariates with control area defined as San Fernando Valley only.

Model 3 = Limited set of covariates with control area defined as San Fernando Valley and Pomona.

Model 4 = Limited set of covariates with control area defined as San Fernando Valley only.

Table F.6

Adjusted Odds Ratios and 95 Percent Confidence Intervals for Patent Ductus Arteriosus for All Variables in Four Logistic Regression Models

Variable	Model 1 (N = 159,850)			Model 2 (N = 145,718)			Model 3 (N = 159,850)			Model 4 (N = 145,718)		
		95% CI			95% CI			95% CI			95% CI	
	OR	Lower	Upper	OR	Lower	Upper	OR	Lower	Upper	OR	Lower	Upper
INTERCEPT	0.00	0.00	0.00	0.00	0.00	0.00	0.00	0.00	0.00	0.00	0.00	0.00
B_YR90	1.15	0.79	1.68	1.21	0.82	1.79	1.16	0.79	1.69	1.21	0.82	1.80
B_YR91	0.90	0.64	1.26	0.96	0.68	1.36	0.90	0.64	1.26	0.96	0.68	1.36
B_YR93	0.16	0.08	0.30	0.17	0.09	0.33	0.16	0.08	0.29	0.17	0.09	0.32
BLACK	1.90	0.87	4.17	2.07	0.90	4.75	1.52	0.71	3.24	1.66	0.74	3.74
WHITE	1.69	1.05	2.72	1.72	1.06	2.78	1.35	0.87	2.10	1.38	0.88	2.16
ASIAN	1.77	0.65	4.86	2.02	0.75	5.40	1.48	0.54	4.07	1.63	0.60	4.41
RACEOTH	1.95	0.84	4.53	1.66	0.66	4.15	1.51	0.66	3.46	1.26	0.52	3.10
Y_M_AGE	0.49	0.22	1.07	0.43	0.18	1.01	0.48	0.22	1.05	0.42	0.18	1.02
L_M_AGE	0.98	0.61	1.59	1.05	0.65	1.72	1.05	0.65	1.69	1.11	0.68	1.81
MALE	1.14	0.83	1.56	1.15	0.84	1.60	1.13	0.83	1.56	1.15	0.83	1.60
ELEMSCHL	1.70	1.08	2.67	1.57	0.98	2.51						
COLLPL	0.92	0.59	1.45	0.84	0.53	1.34						
INADCAR2	0.92	0.54	1.57	0.92	0.53	1.59						
EXPLOW	1.34	0.94	1.90	1.26	0.87	1.82	1.35	0.96	1.90	1.28	0.89	1.84
EXPMED	1.03	0.72	1.48	0.96	0.66	1.40	1.03	0.72	1.48	0.97	0.66	1.42
EXPHI	1.14	0.77	1.70	1.08	0.71	1.64	1.12	0.74	1.69	1.07	0.69	1.65
EXPVHI	1.28	0.84	1.97	1.20	0.77	1.87	1.21	0.79	1.84	1.14	0.74	1.77

Model 1 = Full set of covariates with control area defined as San Fernando Valley and Pomona. Results reported in Chapter Four.

Model 2 = Full set of covariates with control area defined as San Fernando Valley only.

Model 3 = Limited set of covariates with control area defined as San Fernando Valley and Pomona.

Model 4 = Limited set of covariates with control area defined as San Fernando Valley only.

Table F.7

Adjusted Odds Ratios and 95 Percent Confidence Intervals for Other Cardiac Defects for
All Variables in Four Logistic Regression Models

| | Model 1 (N = 159,850) | | | Model 2 (N = 145,718) | | | Model 3 (N = 159,850) | | | Model 4 (N = 145,718) | | |
| | | 95% CI | | | 95% CI | | | 95% CI | | | 95% CI | |
Variable	OR	Lower	Upper	OR	Lower	Upper	OR	Lower	Upper	OR	Lower	Upper
INTERCEPT	0.00	0.00	0.00	0.00	0.00	0.00	0.00	0.00	0.00	0.00	0.00	0.00
B_YR90	1.06	0.71	1.60	1.11	0.70	1.74	1.07	0.71	1.62	1.12	0.71	1.76
B_YR91	0.79	0.54	1.15	0.87	0.59	1.29	0.80	0.55	1.16	0.88	0.59	1.30
B_YR93	0.80	0.56	1.13	0.84	0.57	1.23	0.79	0.56	1.12	0.84	0.57	1.23
BLACK	1.28	0.67	2.43	1.75	1.03	3.00	1.25	0.69	2.28	1.71	1.04	2.79
WHITE	1.07	0.64	1.78	1.18	0.70	1.99	1.03	0.65	1.65	1.13	0.70	1.82
ASIAN	0.79	0.34	1.85	0.96	0.43	2.13	0.77	0.32	1.81	0.91	0.40	2.07
RACEOTH	0.96	0.31	2.96	0.88	0.23	3.33	0.95	0.33	2.69	0.84	0.25	2.89
Y_M_AGE	0.94	0.63	1.39	0.87	0.56	1.33	0.95	0.65	1.38	0.88	0.59	1.34
L_M_AGE	1.17	0.77	1.79	1.23	0.81	1.88	1.18	0.77	1.79	1.23	0.80	1.89
MALE	1.55	1.16	2.06	1.61	1.23	2.10	1.55	1.16	2.06	1.61	1.23	2.10
ELEMSCHL	1.04	0.80	1.35	1.03	0.77	1.38						
COLLPL	1.01	0.69	1.49	0.96	0.64	1.45						
INADCAR2	1.51	1.05	2.16	1.49	1.03	2.16						
EXPLOW	0.98	0.65	1.49	1.01	0.66	1.56	0.99	0.65	1.50	1.02	0.66	1.57
EXPMED	0.85	0.58	1.25	0.84	0.57	1.25	0.86	0.58	1.27	0.85	0.57	1.26
EXPHI	1.05	0.73	1.51	1.07	0.72	1.59	1.05	0.73	1.52	1.08	0.72	1.61
EXPVHI	0.80	0.56	1.15	0.82	0.56	1.19	0.79	0.55	1.14	0.81	0.55	1.19

Model 1 = Full set of covariates with control area defined as San Fernando Valley and Pomona. Results reported in Chapter Four.
Model 2 = Full set of covariates with control area defined as San Fernando Valley only.
Model 3 = Limited set of covariates with control area defined as San Fernando Valley and Pomona.
Model 4 = Limited set of covariates with control area defined as San Fernando Valley only.

Table F.8

Adjusted Odds Ratios and 95 Percent Confidence Intervals for Respiratory System Defects for All Variables in Four Logistic Regression Models

Variable	Model 1 (N = 159,850)			Model 2 (N = 145,718)			Model 3 (N = 159,850)			Model 4 (N = 145,718)		
		95% CI			95% CI			95% CI			95% CI	
	OR	Lower	Upper	OR	Lower	Upper	OR	Lower	Upper	OR	Lower	Upper
INTERCEPT	0.00	0.00	0.00	0.00	0.00	0.00	0.00	0.00	0.00	0.00	0.00	0.00
B_YR90	1.47	1.05	2.06	1.48	1.03	2.11	1.47	1.05	2.06	1.48	1.03	2.11
B_YR91	0.97	0.70	1.35	1.01	0.72	1.41	0.97	0.70	1.35	1.01	0.72	1.41
B_YR93	0.71	0.52	0.97	0.72	0.51	1.00	0.71	0.52	0.97	0.72	0.51	1.01
BLACK	1.31	0.82	2.09	1.41	0.82	2.43	1.28	0.80	2.04	1.37	0.81	2.34
WHITE	1.17	0.79	1.74	1.14	0.74	1.77	1.13	0.77	1.65	1.10	0.72	1.66
ASIAN	0.66	0.24	1.78	0.74	0.27	2.00	0.61	0.23	1.63	0.68	0.25	1.80
RACEOTH	1.00	0.49	2.05	1.06	0.51	2.18	0.91	0.47	1.78	0.95	0.48	1.87
Y_M_AGE	0.96	0.68	1.35	0.94	0.65	1.35	1.01	0.73	1.40	0.99	0.70	1.40
L_M_AGE	1.04	0.71	1.53	1.11	0.76	1.63	1.01	0.69	1.48	1.07	0.73	1.58
MALE	1.18	0.95	1.47	1.20	0.96	1.51	1.18	0.95	1.47	1.20	0.96	1.51
ELEMSCHL	0.87	0.64	1.18	0.85	0.63	1.15						
COLLPL	0.77	0.56	1.07	0.75	0.52	1.07						
INADCAR2	1.08	0.69	1.69	1.07	0.66	1.73						
EXPLOW	1.05	0.78	1.42	1.00	0.73	1.37	1.06	0.79	1.43	1.01	0.74	1.38
EXPMED	1.24	0.91	1.70	1.17	0.84	1.63	1.26	0.92	1.73	1.19	0.85	1.66
EXPHI	1.11	0.85	1.45	1.05	0.79	1.40	1.13	0.86	1.47	1.07	0.81	1.41
EXPVHI	1.04	0.76	1.44	0.99	0.71	1.38	1.05	0.76	1.47	1.00	0.71	1.41

Model 1 = Full set of covariates with control area defined as San Fernando Valley and Pomona. Results reported in Chapter Four.
Model 2 = Full set of covariates with control area defined as San Fernando Valley only.
Model 3 = Limited set of covariates with control area defined as San Fernando Valley and Pomona.
Model 4 = Limited set of covariates with control area defined as San Fernando Valley only.

Table F.9

Adjusted Odds Ratios and 95 Percent Confidence Intervals for Cleft Defects for All Variables in Four Logistic Regression Models

Variable	Model 1 (N = 159,850)			Model 2 (N = 145,718)			Model 3 (N = 159,850)			Model 4 (N = 145,718)		
		95% CI			95% CI			95% CI			95% CI	
	OR	Lower	Upper	OR	Lower	Upper	OR	Lower	Upper	OR	Lower	Upper
INTERCEPT	0.00	0.00	0.00	0.00	0.00	0.00	0.00	0.00	0.00	0.00	0.00	0.00
B_YR90	1.15	0.74	1.79	1.15	0.73	1.83	1.15	0.74	1.80	1.16	0.73	1.84
B_YR91	1.11	0.68	1.82	0.98	0.58	1.66	1.11	0.68	1.82	0.99	0.59	1.66
B_YR93	1.03	0.68	1.56	0.98	0.64	1.51	1.03	0.68	1.56	0.98	0.64	1.50
BLACK	0.78	0.32	1.89	0.78	0.28	2.22	0.77	0.33	1.80	0.80	0.29	2.17
WHITE	1.14	0.71	1.84	1.08	0.65	1.79	1.11	0.71	1.73	1.09	0.68	1.74
ASIAN	0.79	0.22	2.78	0.88	0.24	3.19	0.75	0.21	2.64	0.87	0.24	3.11
RACEOTH	0.53	0.11	2.57	0.55	0.11	2.70	0.50	0.11	2.32	0.55	0.12	2.58
Y_M_AGE	0.72	0.45	1.17	0.81	0.51	1.29	0.74	0.46	1.20	0.84	0.53	1.32
L_M_AGE	0.95	0.60	1.53	0.99	0.61	1.62	0.94	0.57	1.54	0.97	0.58	1.62
MALE	1.36	1.01	1.82	1.35	0.99	1.85	1.36	1.01	1.82	1.35	0.99	1.85
ELEMSCHL	0.92	0.60	1.42	0.86	0.55	1.34						
COLLPL	0.86	0.57	1.30	0.93	0.62	1.41						
INADCAR2	1.15	0.68	1.96	1.28	0.75	2.17						
EXPLOW	1.13	0.62	2.07	1.14	0.61	2.10	1.14	0.62	2.08	1.14	0.62	2.11
EXPMED	0.82	0.57	1.17	0.82	0.56	1.20	0.82	0.58	1.17	0.82	0.56	1.20
EXPHI	1.09	0.79	1.51	1.09	0.76	1.54	1.10	0.80	1.52	1.10	0.78	1.55
EXPVHI	1.10	0.80	1.50	1.09	0.78	1.53	1.10	0.80	1.50	1.10	0.79	1.54

Model 1 = Full set of covariates with control area defined as San Fernando Valley and Pomona Results reported in Chapter Four.
Model 2 = Full set of covariates with control area defined as San Fernando Valley only.
Model 3 = Limited set of covariates with control area defined as San Fernando Valley and Pomona.
Model 4 = Limited set of covariates with control area defined as San Fernando Valley only.

Table F.10

Adjusted Odds Ratios and 95 Percent Confidence Intervals for Pyloric Stenosis for All Variables in Four Logistic Regression Models

Variable	Model 1 (N = 159,850)			Model 2 (N = 145,718)			Model 3 (N = 159,850)			Model 4 (N = 145,718)		
		95% CI			95% CI			95% CI			95% CI	
	OR	Lower	Upper	OR	Lower	Upper	OR	Lower	Upper	OR	Lower	Upper
INTERCEPT	0.00	0.00	0.00	0.00	0.00	0.00	0.00	0.00	0.00	0.00	0.00	0.00
B_YR90	1.06	0.67	1.67	1.10	0.68	1.76	1.06	0.67	1.67	1.10	0.68	1.76
B_YR91	1.02	0.76	1.36	1.02	0.75	1.38	1.02	0.76	1.36	1.02	0.75	1.39
B_YR93	1.06	0.78	1.45	1.06	0.76	1.48	1.07	0.78	1.46	1.07	0.76	1.49
BLACK	0.56	0.24	1.31	0.56	0.22	1.41	0.61	0.27	1.37	0.61	0.25	1.48
WHITE	1.30	0.95	1.79	1.27	0.91	1.78	1.40	1.02	1.91	1.37	0.98	1.91
ASIAN	0.83	0.24	2.81	0.93	0.27	3.20	0.86	0.26	2.81	0.96	0.29	3.16
RACEOTH	0.21	0.03	1.64	0.22	0.03	1.74	0.22	0.03	1.70	0.23	0.03	1.79
Y_M_AGE	0.89	0.52	1.51	0.92	0.53	1.60	0.93	0.54	1.58	0.97	0.56	1.69
L_M_AGE	0.69	0.38	1.24	0.68	0.37	1.26	0.65	0.37	1.16	0.64	0.35	1.17
MALE	5.59	3.98	7.86	5.86	4.09	8.40	5.59	3.98	7.86	5.86	4.09	8.40
ELEMSCHL	0.67	0.47	0.96	0.63	0.43	0.92						
COLLPL	0.90	0.63	1.28	0.87	0.60	1.28						
INADCAR2	1.14	0.67	1.92	1.21	0.72	2.04						
EXPLOW	1.03	0.78	1.35	0.95	0.72	1.25	1.03	0.78	1.36	0.95	0.72	1.26
EXPMED	0.94	0.71	1.26	0.87	0.65	1.16	0.95	0.72	1.26	0.88	0.66	1.17
EXPHI	0.77	0.53	1.13	0.71	0.48	1.04	0.79	0.55	1.14	0.73	0.50	1.06
EXPVHI	1.09	0.82	1.45	1.00	0.75	1.34	1.13	0.85	1.51	1.05	0.78	1.40

Model 1 = Full set of covariates with control area defined as San Fernando Valley and Pomona Results reported in Chapter Four.
Model 2 = Full set of covariates with control area defined as San Fernando Valley only.
Model 3 = Limited set of covariates with control area defined as San Fernando Valley and Pomona.
Model 4 = Limited set of covariates with control area defined as San Fernando Valley only.

Table F.11

Adjusted Odds Ratios and 95 Percent Confidence Intervals for Intestinal Atresias for All Variables in Four Logistic Regression Models

Variable	Model 1 (N = 159,850)			Model 2 (N = 145,718)			Model 3 (N = 159,850)			Model 4 (N = 145,718)		
		95% CI			95% CI			95% CI			95% CI	
	OR	Lower	Upper	OR	Lower	Upper	OR	Lower	Upper	OR	Lower	Upper
INTERCEPT	0.00	0.00	0.00	0.00	0.00	0.00	0.00	0.00	0.00	0.00	0.00	0.00
B_YR90	1.55	0.80	2.99	1.30	0.65	2.62	1.55	0.80	3.00	1.30	0.65	2.61
B_YR91	0.94	0.49	1.81	0.86	0.44	1.70	0.94	0.49	1.81	0.86	0.44	1.69
B_YR93	1.46	0.84	2.54	1.39	0.78	2.48	1.45	0.84	2.51	1.38	0.78	2.46
BLACK	1.54	0.53	4.43	2.10	0.76	5.76	1.33	0.46	3.83	1.82	0.67	4.99
WHITE	1.60	0.95	2.68	1.75	1.04	2.97	1.38	0.85	2.25	1.52	0.93	2.49
ASIAN	1.54	0.53	4.45	1.33	0.32	5.58	1.39	0.48	4.05	1.15	0.29	4.59
Y_M_AGE	1.44	0.82	2.52	1.62	0.93	2.81	1.39	0.80	2.41	1.62	0.96	2.74
L_M_AGE	1.32	0.65	2.68	1.45	0.68	3.10	1.40	0.70	2.82	1.49	0.70	3.17
MALE	1.49	1.05	2.13	1.48	1.00	2.19	1.49	1.05	2.13	1.48	1.00	2.19
ELEMSCHL	1.57	1.03	2.38	1.37	0.89	2.09						
COLLPL	1.04	0.58	1.86	0.85	0.48	1.50						
INADCAR2	0.91	0.42	1.97	0.77	0.31	1.94						
EXPLOW	1.04	0.62	1.74	1.09	0.62	1.89	1.04	0.62	1.74	1.09	0.63	1.91
EXPMED	0.85	0.54	1.34	0.84	0.51	1.38	0.84	0.54	1.33	0.84	0.51	1.39
EXPHI	1.15	0.83	1.58	1.17	0.81	1.68	1.12	0.82	1.54	1.16	0.81	1.67
EXPVHI	0.71	0.42	1.21	0.72	0.41	1.28	0.68	0.40	1.14	0.70	0.40	1.23

Model 1 = Full set of covariates with control area defined as San Fernando Valley and Pomona. Results reported in Chapter Four.
Model 2 = Full set of covariates with control area defined as San Fernando Valley only.
Model 3 = Limited set of covariates with control area defined as San Fernando Valley and Pomona.
Model 4 = Limited set of covariates with control area defined as San Fernando Valley only.

Table F.12

Adjusted Odds Ratios and 95 Percent Confidence Intervals for Other Digestive System Defects for All Variables in Four Logistic Regression Models

Variable	Model 1 (N = 159,850)			Model 2 (N = 145,718)			Model 3 (N = 159,850)			Model 4 (N = 145,718)		
		95% CI			95% CI			95% CI			95% CI	
	OR	Lower	Upper	OR	Lower	Upper	OR	Lower	Upper	OR	Lower	Upper
INTERCEPT	0.00	0.00	0.00	0.00	0.00	0.00	0.00	0.00	0.00	0.00	0.00	0.00
B_YR90	1.29	0.99	1.67	1.25	0.96	1.64	1.29	1.00	1.68	1.26	0.96	1.65
B_YR91	0.92	0.73	1.16	0.93	0.73	1.18	0.92	0.73	1.16	0.93	0.73	1.19
B_YR93	0.90	0.70	1.17	0.89	0.68	1.18	0.90	0.70	1.17	0.89	0.68	1.17
BLACK	0.92	0.52	1.62	0.86	0.44	1.67	0.89	0.49	1.61	0.83	0.42	1.62
WHITE	1.48	1.13	1.92	1.47	1.11	1.94	1.42	1.14	1.77	1.40	1.11	1.77
ASIAN	0.99	0.47	2.08	0.95	0.40	2.22	0.93	0.44	1.97	0.88	0.38	2.05
RACEOTH	0.84	0.39	1.82	0.73	0.32	1.67	0.78	0.36	1.68	0.68	0.29	1.55
Y_M_AGE	1.35	0.97	1.88	1.37	0.97	1.94	1.39	1.03	1.88	1.41	1.03	1.93
L_M_AGE	0.91	0.65	1.30	0.94	0.66	1.35	0.90	0.64	1.28	0.93	0.65	1.33
MALE	1.25	1.01	1.54	1.25	1.00	1.57	1.25	1.01	1.54	1.25	1.00	1.57
ELEMSCHL	0.97	0.73	1.29	0.97	0.73	1.29						
COLLPL	0.86	0.63	1.17	0.85	0.61	1.18						
INADCAR2	1.12	0.76	1.66	1.12	0.75	1.68						
EXPLOW	1.20	0.86	1.68	1.12	0.81	1.57	1.21	0.86	1.69	1.13	0.81	1.58
EXPMED	1.40	1.15	1.72	1.33	1.08	1.62	1.42	1.16	1.73	1.34	1.09	1.64
EXPHI	1.11	0.91	1.37	1.05	0.86	1.28	1.12	0.92	1.38	1.06	0.87	1.29
EXPVHI	1.07	0.75	1.53	1.01	0.71	1.42	1.07	0.74	1.55	1.01	0.70	1.44

Model 1 = Full set of covariates with control area defined as San Fernando Valley and Pomona Results reported in Chapter Four.

Model 2 = Full set of covariates with control area defined as San Fernando Valley only.

Model 3 = Limited set of covariates with control area defined as San Fernando Valley and Pomona.

Model 4 = Limited set of covariates with control area defined as San Fernando Valley only.

Table F.13

Adjusted Odds Ratios and 95 Percent Confidence Intervals for Urogenital System Defects for All Variables in Four Logistic Regression Models

Variable	Model 1 (N = 159,850)			Model 2 (N = 145,718)			Model 3 (N = 159,850)			Model 4 (N = 145,718)		
	OR	95% CI Lower	Upper	OR	95% CI Lower	Upper	OR	95% CI Lower	Upper	OR	95% CI Lower	Upper
INTERCEPT	0.00	0.00	0.00	0.00	0.00	0.00	0.00	0.00	0.00	0.00	0.00	0.00
B_YR90	1.17	0.92	1.50	1.09	0.85	1.39	1.17	0.92	1.50	1.09	0.85	1.39
B_YR91	0.99	0.75	1.29	0.99	0.74	1.31	0.99	0.75	1.29	0.99	0.74	1.31
B_YR93	0.95	0.74	1.22	0.94	0.72	1.23	0.95	0.74	1.22	0.94	0.72	1.23
BLACK	1.51	1.10	2.07	1.37	0.96	1.97	1.66	1.20	2.31	1.50	1.05	2.15
WHITE	1.67	1.40	2.01	1.69	1.40	2.04	1.87	1.55	2.25	1.86	1.54	2.26
ASIAN	0.97	0.50	1.90	0.79	0.38	1.63	1.11	0.58	2.12	0.90	0.46	1.77
RACEOTH	1.19	0.69	2.05	1.25	0.73	2.14	1.42	0.83	2.42	1.47	0.86	2.51
Y_M_AGE	1.11	0.86	1.44	1.07	0.82	1.40	1.06	0.82	1.37	1.02	0.78	1.33
L_M_AGE	0.90	0.63	1.29	0.86	0.60	1.24	0.91	0.65	1.28	0.87	0.61	1.25
MALE	3.12	2.48	3.92	3.06	2.41	3.88	3.12	2.48	3.92	3.06	2.41	3.88
ELEMSCHL	0.92	0.73	1.17	0.97	0.77	1.23						
COLLPL	1.31	1.02	1.70	1.32	1.00	1.75						
INADCAR2	1.05	0.71	1.54	1.03	0.69	1.55						
EXPLOW	1.18	0.97	1.45	1.11	0.90	1.35	1.17	0.96	1.43	1.09	0.89	1.34
EXPMED	1.03	0.70	1.52	0.97	0.66	1.44	1.02	0.69	1.51	0.96	0.64	1.42
EXPHI	0.91	0.72	1.14	0.85	0.67	1.07	0.90	0.71	1.13	0.84	0.66	1.05
EXPVHI	0.98	0.73	1.31	0.92	0.68	1.23	0.99	0.73	1.34	0.92	0.68	1.25

Model 1 = Full set of covariates with control area defined as San Fernando Valley and Pomona Results reported in Chapter Four.
Model 2 = Full set of covariates with control area defined as San Fernando Valley only.
Model 3 = Limited set of covariates with control area defined as San Fernando Valley and Pomona.
Model 4 = Limited set of covariates with control area defined as San Fernando Valley only.

Table F.14

Adjusted Odds Ratios and 95 Percent Confidence Intervals for Limb Defects for All Variables in Four Logistic Regression Models

Variable	Model 1 (N = 159,850)			Model 2 (N = 145,718)			Model 3 (N = 159,850)			Model 4 (N = 145,718)		
		95% CI			95% CI			95% CI			95% CI	
	OR	Lower	Upper	OR	Lower	Upper	OR	Lower	Upper	OR	Lower	Upper
INTERCEPT	0.00	0.00	0.00	0.00	0.00	0.00	0.00	0.00	0.00	0.00	0.00	0.00
B_YR90	1.73	0.56	5.34	1.73	0.56	5.35	1.78	0.58	5.39	1.76	0.58	5.37
B_YR91	1.45	0.59	3.55	1.45	0.59	3.57	1.48	0.61	3.58	1.48	0.61	3.59
B_YR93	1.78	0.60	5.23	1.58	0.52	4.84	1.75	0.59	5.15	1.55	0.51	4.76
NONHISP	0.49	0.22	1.11	0.53	0.23	1.21	0.45	0.21	0.97	0.47	0.22	1.03
Y_M_AGE	1.65	0.83	3.28	1.59	0.77	3.28	1.66	0.84	3.27	1.58	0.77	3.23
L_M_AGE	1.09	0.46	2.58	1.10	0.46	2.61	1.14	0.48	2.69	1.17	0.49	2.76
MALE	1.34	0.66	2.71	1.36	0.66	2.81	1.34	0.66	2.70	1.36	0.66	2.80
ELEMSCHL	1.29	0.72	2.30	1.40	0.77	2.54						
COLLPL	1.12	0.49	2.53	1.15	0.50	2.63						
INADCAR2	2.26	1.10	4.62	2.07	0.97	4.44						
EXPLOW	1.02	0.47	2.22	0.93	0.43	1.98	1.04	0.47	2.27	0.94	0.44	2.02
EXPMED	0.99	0.45	2.15	0.89	0.41	1.92	1.00	0.45	2.22	0.89	0.40	1.98
EXPHI	2.08	1.48	2.91	1.87	1.40	2.48	2.07	1.47	2.91	1.85	1.38	2.47
EXPVHI	1.38	0.79	2.44	1.25	0.73	2.14	1.32	0.77	2.26	1.19	0.72	1.96

Model 1 = Full set of covariates with control area defined as San Fernando Valley and Pomona Results reported in Chapter Four.

Model 2 = Full set of covariates with control area defined as San Fernando Valley only.

Model 3 = Limited set of covariates with control area defined as San Fernando Valley and Pomona.

Model 4 = Limited set of covariates with control area defined as San Fernando Valley only.

Table F.15

Adjusted Odds Ratios and 95 Percent Confidence Intervals for Other Musculoskeletal Defects for All Variables in Four Logistic Regression Models

Variable	Model 1 (N = 159,850)			Model 2 (N = 145,718)			Model 3 (N = 159,850)			Model 4 (N = 145,718)		
	OR	95% CI Lower	Upper	OR	95% CI Lower	Upper	OR	95% CI Lower	Upper	OR	95% CI Lower	Upper
INTERCEPT	0.01	0.00	0.01	0.01	0.00	0.01	0.01	0.00	0.01	0.01	0.00	0.01
B_YR90	1.33	1.07	1.66	1.38	1.10	1.73	1.33	1.07	1.66	1.38	1.10	1.72
B_YR91	0.91	0.78	1.07	0.91	0.76	1.08	0.91	0.78	1.07	0.91	0.76	1.08
B_YR93	0.85	0.72	1.02	0.86	0.71	1.04	0.85	0.72	1.02	0.86	0.71	1.04
BLACK	1.34	1.00	1.80	1.43	1.02	1.99	1.33	1.02	1.74	1.40	1.03	1.90
WHITE	1.20	0.99	1.46	1.19	0.97	1.46	1.19	1.00	1.42	1.16	0.97	1.40
ASIAN	1.26	0.74	2.12	1.25	0.68	2.28	1.25	0.74	2.10	1.22	0.67	2.22
RACEOTH	0.83	0.51	1.33	0.82	0.50	1.37	0.82	0.52	1.29	0.80	0.49	1.29
Y_M_AGE	1.21	0.99	1.48	1.23	1.00	1.52	1.21	0.99	1.49	1.24	1.00	1.53
L_M_AGE	1.06	0.82	1.37	1.07	0.82	1.41	1.06	0.82	1.37	1.08	0.82	1.41
MALE	1.11	1.00	1.23	1.11	1.00	1.24	1.11	1.00	1.23	1.11	1.00	1.24
ELEMSCHL	1.02	0.87	1.19	1.03	0.89	1.21						
COLLPL	1.00	0.82	1.22	0.96	0.79	1.18						
INADCAR2	1.01	0.80	1.28	0.99	0.76	1.27						
EXPLOW	0.84	0.66	1.06	0.77	0.62	0.97	0.84	0.66	1.06	0.78	0.62	0.97
EXPMED	1.16	0.93	1.44	1.07	0.87	1.32	1.16	0.93	1.43	1.07	0.87	1.32
EXPHI	1.01	0.81	1.26	0.94	0.75	1.17	1.01	0.81	1.26	0.94	0.76	1.16
EXPVHI	0.93	0.72	1.20	0.87	0.67	1.12	0.93	0.72	1.20	0.86	0.67	1.11

Model 1 = Full set of covariates with control area defined as San Fernando Valley and Pomona Results reported in Chapter Four.

Model 2 = Full set of covariates with control area defined as San Fernando Valley only.

Model 3 = Limited set of covariates with control area defined as San Fernando Valley and Pomona.

Model 4 = Limited set of covariates with control area defined as San Fernando Valley only.

Table F.16

Adjusted Odds Ratios and 95 Percent Confidence Intervals for Integument Defects for All Variables in Four Logistic Regression Models

| Variable | Model 1 (N = 159,850) | | | Model 2 (N = 145,718) | | | Model 3 (N = 159,850) | | | Model 4 (N = 145,718) | | |
| | | 95% CI | | | 95% CI | | | 95% CI | | | 95% CI | |
	OR	Lower	Upper	OR	Lower	Upper	OR	Lower	Upper	OR	Lower	Upper
INTERCEPT	0.00	0.00	0.00	0.00	0.00	0.00	0.00	0.00	0.00	0.00	0.00	0.00
B_YR90	0.99	0.75	1.30	0.98	0.74	1.30	0.99	0.76	1.30	0.99	0.75	1.31
B_YR91	0.93	0.74	1.16	0.91	0.72	1.15	0.93	0.74	1.17	0.91	0.72	1.15
B_YR93	0.67	0.54	0.83	0.68	0.54	0.84	0.67	0.54	0.83	0.67	0.54	0.83
BLACK	0.93	0.50	1.74	1.19	0.68	2.09	0.84	0.47	1.48	1.03	0.62	1.74
WHITE	0.98	0.72	1.35	1.02	0.73	1.42	0.88	0.64	1.20	0.88	0.63	1.22
ASIAN	0.99	0.52	1.88	1.02	0.49	2.11	0.89	0.47	1.68	0.87	0.43	1.78
RACEOTH	1.34	0.80	2.26	1.44	0.87	2.40	1.16	0.70	1.93	1.19	0.71	1.98
Y_M_AGE	0.99	0.71	1.38	0.98	0.69	1.38	1.00	0.73	1.38	0.99	0.71	1.39
L_M_AGE	0.93	0.67	1.30	0.91	0.64	1.29	0.96	0.69	1.32	0.94	0.67	1.32
MALE	1.18	1.00	1.39	1.18	0.99	1.40	1.18	1.00	1.39	1.18	0.99	1.40
ELEMSCHL	1.23	0.99	1.53	1.29	1.06	1.57						
COLLPL	0.88	0.70	1.12	0.84	0.66	1.06						
INADCAR2	1.11	0.78	1.56	1.07	0.74	1.53						
EXPLOW	0.69	0.49	0.99	0.61	0.44	0.87	0.70	0.49	1.00	0.62	0.44	0.88
EXPMED	1.13	0.74	1.75	0.99	0.65	1.49	1.14	0.74	1.75	0.99	0.66	1.50
EXPHI	0.74	0.52	1.05	0.65	0.47	0.92	0.74	0.52	1.04	0.65	0.46	0.91
EXPVHI	0.71	0.48	1.06	0.64	0.43	0.94	0.69	0.47	1.02	0.61	0.42	0.90

Model 1 = Full set of covariates with control area defined as San Fernando Valley and Pomona Results reported in Chapter Four.

Model 2 = Full set of covariates with control area defined as San Fernando Valley only.

Model 3 = Limited set of covariates with control area defined as San Fernando Valley and Pomona.

Model 4 = Limited set of covariates with control area defined as San Fernando Valley only.

Table F.17

Adjusted Odds Ratios and 95 Percent Confidence Intervals for All Other Defects for All Variables in Four Logistic Regression Models

Variable	Model 1 (N = 159,850)			Model 2 (N = 145,718)			Model 3 (N = 159,850)			Model 4 (N = 145,718)		
		95% CI			95% CI			95% CI			95% CI	
	OR	Lower	Upper	OR	Lower	Upper	OR	Lower	Upper	OR	Lower	Upper
INTERCEPT	0.00	0.00	0.00	0.00	0.00	0.00	0.00	0.00	0.00	0.00	0.00	0.00
B_YR90	1.64	0.58	4.62	1.78	0.61	5.21	1.67	0.59	4.73	1.81	0.61	5.32
B_YR91	1.29	0.54	3.11	1.41	0.56	3.53	1.31	0.54	3.17	1.43	0.57	3.61
B_YR93	1.78	0.73	4.33	1.75	0.69	4.44	1.76	0.73	4.26	1.74	0.69	4.39
BLACK	1.01	0.22	4.58	1.33	0.31	5.77	0.98	0.23	4.15	1.26	0.31	5.16
WHITE	0.68	0.22	2.09	0.74	0.24	2.29	0.63	0.23	1.74	0.67	0.24	1.85
ASIAN	0.92	0.11	7.68	1.09	0.13	9.27	0.84	0.11	6.33	0.93	0.12	7.03
RACEOTH	1.75	0.39	7.84	1.97	0.44	8.85	1.63	0.35	7.50	1.71	0.36	7.98
Y_M_AGE	1.62	0.98	2.68	1.56	0.92	2.65	1.71	1.08	2.72	1.68	1.04	2.72
L_M_AGE	1.23	0.48	3.15	1.29	0.50	3.33	1.21	0.46	3.18	1.26	0.48	3.34
MALE	0.96	0.52	1.77	1.00	0.53	1.87	0.96	0.52	1.77	1.00	0.53	1.87
ELEMSCHL	0.94	0.44	2.02	0.92	0.41	2.07						
COLLPL	0.87	0.37	2.05	0.74	0.30	1.83						
INADCAR2	2.07	0.98	4.36	1.93	0.87	4.30						
EXPLOW	2.05	1.09	3.83	1.92	1.04	3.55	2.08	1.12	3.88	1.96	1.07	3.60
EXPMED	0.66	0.24	1.80	0.60	0.21	1.68	0.67	0.25	1.85	0.61	0.22	1.72
EXPHI	1.56	0.71	3.44	1.44	0.66	3.15	1.59	0.73	3.47	1.47	0.68	3.18
EXPVHI	0.84	0.37	1.92	0.79	0.35	1.79	0.84	0.36	1.97	0.78	0.33	1.84

Model 1 = Full set of covariates with control area defined as San Fernando Valley and Pomona Results reported in Chapter Four.

Model 2 = Full set of covariates with control area defined as San Fernando Valley only.

Model 3 = Limited set of covariates with control area defined as San Fernando Valley and Pomona.

Model 4 = Limited set of covariates with control area defined as San Fernando Valley only.

Table F.18

Adjusted Odds Ratios and 95 Percent Confidence Intervals for Chromosomal Syndromes for All Variables in Four Logistic Regression Models

Variable	Model 1 (N = 160,328)			Model 2 (N = 146,165)			Model 3 (N = 160,328)			Model 4 (N = 146,165)		
		95% CI			95% CI			95% CI			95% CI	
	OR	Lower	Upper	OR	Lower	Upper	OR	Lower	Upper	OR	Lower	Upper
INTERCEPT	0.00	0.00	0.00	0.00	0.00	0.00	0.00	0.00	0.00	0.00	0.00	0.00
B_YR90	1.10	0.76	1.61	1.15	0.77	1.71	1.11	0.76	1.61	1.16	0.78	1.72
B_YR91	0.99	0.75	1.31	0.99	0.74	1.34	0.99	0.75	1.32	0.99	0.73	1.35
B_YR93	1.07	0.83	1.39	1.07	0.82	1.41	1.06	0.82	1.38	1.07	0.81	1.40
BLACK	0.85	0.42	1.70	0.73	0.36	1.48	0.78	0.39	1.54	0.67	0.34	1.32
WHITE	0.90	0.61	1.33	0.84	0.55	1.26	0.84	0.62	1.14	0.78	0.57	1.07
ASIAN	0.66	0.32	1.34	0.49	0.20	1.20	0.64	0.33	1.25	0.48	0.21	1.13
RACEOTH	0.97	0.48	1.95	1.01	0.50	2.05	0.95	0.48	1.88	1.00	0.50	1.97
Y_M_AGE	0.78	0.49	1.24	0.81	0.50	1.30	0.73	0.47	1.13	0.75	0.48	1.18
L_M_AGE	3.33	2.53	4.40	3.18	2.39	4.25	3.58	2.79	4.60	3.42	2.64	4.45
MALE	1.06	0.82	1.36	1.14	0.88	1.46	1.06	0.82	1.36	1.14	0.88	1.46
ELEMSCHL	1.53	1.08	2.16	1.55	1.08	2.22						
COLLPL	1.30	0.86	1.98	1.29	0.83	2.02						
INADCAR2	1.06	0.69	1.62	0.96	0.61	1.51						
EXPLOW	0.69	0.48	0.98	0.65	0.45	0.93	0.69	0.48	0.98	0.65	0.45	0.93
EXPMED	1.10	0.78	1.55	1.06	0.75	1.51	1.09	0.78	1.53	1.05	0.74	1.49
EXPHI	1.09	0.86	1.37	1.04	0.81	1.32	1.06	0.83	1.36	1.01	0.78	1.30
EXPVHI	1.13	0.81	1.58	1.08	0.77	1.52	1.08	0.78	1.50	1.04	0.74	1.44

Model 1 = Full set of covariates with control area defined as San Fernando Valley and Pomona Results reported in Chapter Four.

Model 2 = Full set of covariates with control area defined as San Fernando Valley only.

Model 3 = Limited set of covariates with control area defined as San Fernando Valley and Pomona.

Model 4 = Limited set of covariates with control area defined as San Fernando Valley only.

Table F.19

Adjusted Odds Ratios and 95 Percent Confidence Intervals for Syndromes Other than Chromosomal for All Variables in Four Logistic Regression Models

Variable	Model 1 (N = 160,328)			Model 2 (N = 146,165)			Model 3 (N = 160,328)			Model 4 (N = 146,165)		
		95% CI			95% CI			95% CI			95% CI	
	OR	Lower	Upper	OR	Lower	Upper	OR	Lower	Upper	OR	Lower	Upper
INTERCEPT	0.00	0.00	0.00	0.00	0.00	0.00	0.00	0.00	0.00	0.00	0.00	0.00
B_YR90	1.11	0.71	1.73	1.14	0.72	1.80	1.11	0.71	1.74	1.14	0.72	1.81
B_YR91	1.17	0.76	1.80	1.16	0.73	1.85	1.18	0.77	1.81	1.17	0.74	1.85
B_YR93	1.14	0.73	1.80	1.23	0.78	1.94	1.14	0.72	1.79	1.23	0.78	1.94
BLACK	1.29	0.62	2.68	0.95	0.37	2.42	1.20	0.60	2.38	0.91	0.36	2.26
WHITE	0.70	0.42	1.18	0.65	0.39	1.09	0.64	0.43	0.96	0.61	0.40	0.92
ASIAN	0.58	0.07	4.68	0.61	0.08	4.92	0.51	0.07	4.00	0.55	0.07	4.30
RACEOTH	0.30	0.04	2.04	0.29	0.04	1.95	0.25	0.03	1.89	0.26	0.03	1.91
Y_M_AGE	0.78	0.58	1.04	0.74	0.56	0.98	0.82	0.60	1.12	0.78	0.57	1.06
L_M_AGE	0.93	0.52	1.68	0.90	0.49	1.65	0.92	0.53	1.60	0.88	0.50	1.56
MALE	1.17	0.82	1.66	1.15	0.80	1.67	1.17	0.82	1.66	1.15	0.80	1.67
ELEMSCHL	0.96	0.63	1.47	0.93	0.60	1.44	.	.	.	.	.	.
COLLPL	0.74	0.45	1.21	0.79	0.48	1.29	.	.	.	.	.	.
INADCAR2	1.25	0.84	1.85	1.25	0.83	1.88	.	.	.	.	.	.
EXPLOW	1.17	0.69	1.99	1.03	0.61	1.72	1.18	0.69	2.01	1.04	0.62	1.74
EXPMED	0.88	0.64	1.20	0.80	0.59	1.08	0.89	0.65	1.22	0.81	0.59	1.10
EXPHI	1.01	0.68	1.50	0.90	0.62	1.31	1.02	0.69	1.51	0.91	0.63	1.32
EXPVHI	0.89	0.53	1.48	0.78	0.48	1.28	0.88	0.53	1.46	0.78	0.48	1.27

Model 1 = Full set of covariates with control area defined as San Fernando Valley and Pomona Results reported in Chapter Four.
Model 2 = Full set of covariates with control area defined as San Fernando Valley only.
Model 3 = Limited set of covariates with control area defined as San Fernando Valley and Pomona.
Model 4 = Limited set of covariates with control area defined as San Fernando Valley only.

BIBLIOGRAPHY

Ames, B. N., "Dietary Carcinogens and Anticarcinogens, Oxygen Radicals and Degenerative Diseases," *Science*, 221, 1983, pp. 1256–1264.

Arbuckle, T. E., G. J. Sherman, P. N. Corey, et al., "Water Nitrates and Central Nervous System Birth Defects: A Population Based Case Control Study," *Archives of Environmental Health*, 43(2), 1988, pp. 162–167.

Aschengrau, A., S. Zierler, and A. Cohen, "Quality of Community Drinking Water and the Occurrence of Spontaneous Abortion," *Archives of Environmental Health*, 44(5), 1989, pp. 283–290.

Aschengrau, A., et al., "Quality of Community Drinking Water and the Occurrence of Late Adverse Pregnancy Outcomes," *Archives of Environmental Health*, 48(2), 1993, pp. 105–113.

Barros, H., M. Tavares, and T. Rodrigues, "Role of Prenatal Care in Preterm Birth and Low Birth Weight in Portugal," *Journal of Public Health Medicine*, 18(3), 1996, pp. 321–328.

Berkowitz, G. S., and E. Papiernik, "Epidemiology of Preterm Birth," *Epidemiologic Reviews*, 15(2), 1993, pp. 414–443.

Berry, M., and F. Bove, "Birth Weight Reduction Associated with Residence Near a Hazardous Waste Landfill," *Environmental Health Perspectives*, 15(8), 1997, pp. 856–861.

Bhopal, R. S., P. Phillimore, S. Moffatt, and C. Foy, "Is Living Near a Coking Works Harmful to Health? A Study of Industrial Air Pollution," *Journal of Epidemiology and Community Health*, 48(3), 1994, pp. 237–247.

Bianchi, F., D. Cianciulli, A. Pierini, et al., "Congenital Malformations and Maternal Occupation: A Registry Based Case-Control Study," *Occupational and Environmental Medicine*, 54(4), 1997, pp. 223–228.

Blanton, M., *The Layperson's Guide to Water Recycling and Reuse*, Sacramento, Calif.: Water Education Foundation, 1992.

Bookman-Edmonston Engineering, Inc., *Engineering Background Studies for RAND Corporation's Health Effects Study*, Glendale, Calif., May 1993.

Bookman-Edmonston Engineering, Inc., *Addendum to Engineering Background Studies for RAND Corporation's Health Effects Study*, Glendale, Calif., April 1998.

Bound, J. P., P. W. Harvey, D. M. Brookes, et al., "The Incidence of Anencephalus in the Fylde Peninsula 1956–76 and Changes in Water Hardness," *Journal of Epidemiology and Community Health*, 35, 1981, pp. 102–105.

Bove, F. J., M. C. Fulcomer, J. B. Klotz, et al., "Public Drinking Water Contamination and Birth Outcomes," *American Journal of Epidemiology*, 141(9), 1995, pp. 850–862.

Breslow, N. E., and D. G. Clayton, "Approximate Inference in Generalized Mixed Models," *Journal of the American Statistical Association*, 88(421), 1993, pp. 9–25.

British Paediatric Association, *British Paediatric Association Classification of Diseases: Perinatal Supplement: Codes Designed for Use in the Classification of Perinatal Disorders*, London: The Association, 1979.

Byrne, J., D. Warburton, J. Kline, W. Blanc, and Z. Stein, "Morphology of Early Fetal Deaths and Their Chromosomal Characteristics," *Teratology*, 32, 1985, pp. 297–315.

Canfield, M. A., J. F. Annegers, J. D. Brender, S. P. Cooper, and F. Greenberg, "Hispanic Origin and Neural Tube Defects in Houston/Harris County, Texas. I. Descriptive Epidemiology," *American Journal of Epidemiology*, 143(1), 1996, pp. 1–11.

Carter, C. O., and K. S. Evans, "Spina Bifida and Anencephalus in Greater London," *Journal of Medical Genetics*, 10, 1973, pp. 209–234.

Census of Population and Housing, 1990: Summary Tape File 1 (California) [machine-readable data files]/prepared by the Bureau of the Census, Washington, D.C., 1991a.

Census of Population and Housing, 1990: Summary Tape File 2 (California) [machine-readable data files]/prepared by the Bureau of the Census, Washington, D.C., 1991b.

Census of Population and Housing, 1990: Summary Tape File 3 (California) [machine-readable data files]/prepared by the Bureau of the Census, Washington, D.C., 1991c.

Centers for Disease Control and Prevention, "Spina Bifida Incidence at Birth—United States, 1983–1990," *Morbidity and Mortality Weekly Report*, 41, 1992, pp. 497–500.

Centers for Disease Control and Prevention, "Down's Syndrome Prevalence at Birth—United States, 1983–1990," *Morbidity and Mortality Weekly Report*, 43, 1994, pp. 617–622.

Ceron-Mireles, P., C. I. Sanchez-Carrillo, S. D. Harlow, and R. M. Nunez-Urquiza, "Conditions of Maternal Work and Low Birth Weight in Mexico City," *Salud Publica de Mexico,* 39(1), 1997, pp. 2–10.

Chen, A. T. L., and L. Sever, "Re: Public Drinking Water Contamination and Birth Outcomes," Letter to the Editor, *American Journal of Epidemiology,* 143(11), 1996, pp. 1179–1180.

Cobas, J. A., H. Balcazar, M. B. Benin, V. M. Keith, and Y. Chong, "Acculturation and Low-Birth Weight Infants Among Latino Women: A Reanalysis of HHANES Data with Structural Equation Models," *American Journal of Public Health,* 86(3), 1996, pp. 394–396.

Cogswell, M. E., and R. Yip, "The Influence of Fetal and Maternal Factors on the Distribution of Birth Weight," *Seminars in Perinatology,* 19(3), 1995, pp. 222–240.

Cohn, P. D., J. A. Fagliano, and J. B. Klotz, "Assessing Human Health Effects from Chemical Contaminants in Drinking Water," *New Jersey Medicine,* 91(10), 1994, pp. 719–722.

Cordier, S., M. C. Ha, S. Ayme, and J. Goujard, "Maternal Occupational Exposure and Congenital Malformations," *Scandinavian Journal of Work, Environment and Health,* 18(1), 1992, pp. 11–17.

Correa, A., R. H. Gray, R. Cohen, N. Rothman, F. Shah, H. Seacat, and M. Corn, "Ethylene Glycol Ethers and Risks of Spontaneous Abortion and Subfertility," *American Journal of Epidemiology,* 143(7), 1996, pp. 707–717.

Cragan, J. D., H. E. Roberts, L. D. Edmonds, et al., "Surveillance for Anencephaly and Spina Bifida and the Impact of Prenatal Diagnosis—United States, 1985–1994," *MMWR CDC Surveillance Summary,* 44, 1995, pp. 1–13.

Cramer, J. C., "Racial and Ethnic Differences in Birth Weight: The Role of Income and Financial Assistance," *Demography,* 32(2), 1995, pp. 231–247.

Craun, G. F., "Epidemiology Studies of Water Disinfectants and Disinfection By-Products," in G. F. Craun, ed., *Safety of Water Disinfection: Balancing Chemical and Microbial Risks,* Washington, D.C.: ILSI Press, 1993, pp. 277–301.

Croen, L. A., G. M. Shaw, N. G. Jenswold, et al., "Birth Defects Monitoring in California: A Resource for Epidemiological Research," *Paediatric and Perinatal Epidemiology,* 5, 1991, pp. 423–427.

Croen, L. A., G. M. Shaw, L. Sanbonatsu, S. Selvin, and P. A. Buffler, "Maternal Residential Proximity to Hazardous Waste Sites and Risk for Selected Congenital Malformations," *Epidemiology,* 8, 1997, pp. 347–354.

Crook, J., T. Asano, and M. Nellor, "Groundwater Recharge with Reclaimed Water in California," *Water Environment and Technology,* 2(8), 1990, pp. 42–49.

Davis, J. C., and M. J. McCullaugh (eds.), *Display and Analysis of Spatial Data,* New York: John Wiley and Sons, 1975.

Deane, M., S. H. Swan, J. A. Harris, D. M. Epstein, and R. R. Neutra, "Adverse Pregnancy Outcomes in Relation to Water Consumption: A Re-Analysis of Data from the Original Santa Clara County Study, California, 1980–1981," *Epidemiology*, 3(2), 1992, pp. 94–97.

Deane, M., S. H. Swan, J. A. Harris, D. M. Epstein, and R. R. Neutra, "Adverse Pregnancy Outcomes in Relation to Water Contamination, Santa Clara County, California, 1980–1981," *American Journal of Epidemiology*, 129(5), 1989, pp. 894–904.

Defo, B. K., and M. Partin, "Determinants of Low Birth Weight: A Comparative Study," *Journal of Biosocial Science*, 25(1), 1993, pp. 87–100.

Dimich-Ward, H., C. Hertzman, K. Teschke, R. Hershler, S. A. Marion, A. Ostry, and S. Kelly, "Reproductive Effects of Paternal Exposure to Chlorophenate Wood Preservatives in the Sawmill Industry," *Scandinavian Journal of Work, Environment and Health*, 22(4), 1996, pp. 267–273.

Dominguez-Rojas, V., J. R. de Juanes-Pardo, P. Astasio-Arbiza, P. Ortega-Molina, and E. Gordillo-Florencio, "Spontaneous Abortion in a Hospital Population: Are Tobacco and Coffee Intake Risk Factors?" *European Journal of Epidemiology*, 10(6), 1994, pp. 665–668.

Dorsch, M. M., R. K. R. Scragg, A. J. McMichael, et al., "Congenital Malformations and Maternal Drinking Water Supply in Rural South Australia: A Case Control Study," *American Journal of Epidemiology*, 119(4), 1984, pp. 473–486.

Druschel, C., J. P. Hughes, and C. Olsen, "Mortality Among Infants with Congenital Malformations, New York State, 1983 to 1988," *Public Health Reports*, 111(4), 1996, pp. 359–365.

Elwood, J. M., and A. J. Coldman, "Water Composition in the Etiology of Anencephalus," *American Journal of Epidemiology*, 113(6), 1981, pp. 681–690.

Eskenazi, B., L. Fenster, S. Wight, P. English, G. C. Windham, and S. H. Swan, "Physical Exertion as a Risk Factor for Spontaneous Abortion," *Epidemiology*, 5(1), 1994, pp. 6–13.

Eskenazi, B., A. W. Prehn, and R. E. Christianson, "Passive and Active Maternal Smoking as Measured by Serum Cotinine: The Effect on Birth Weight," *American Journal of Public Health*, 85(3), 1995, pp. 395–398.

Fedrick, J., "Anencephalus and the Local Water Supply," *Nature* (London), 227, 1970, p. 176.

Fenster, L., C. Schaefer, A. Mathur, R. A. Hiatt, C. Pieper, A. E. Hubbard, J. Van Behren, and S. H. Swan, "Psychological Stress in the Workplace and Spontaneous Abortion," *American Journal of Epidemiology*, 142(11), 1995, pp. 1176–1183.

Fenster, L., G. C. Windham, S. H. Swan, D. M. Epstein, and R. R. Neutra, "Tap or Bottled Water Consumption and Spontaneous Abortion in a Case-Control Study of Reporting Consistency," *Epidemiology*, 3(2), 1992, pp. 120–124.

Fielding, D. W., and R. W. Smithells, "Anencephalus and Water Hardness in South-West Lancashire," *British Journal of Preventive and Social Medicine,* 25, 1971, pp. 217–219.

Forrester, M. B., R. D. Merz, and P. W. Yoon "Impact of Prenatal Diagnosis and Elective Termination on the Prevalence of Selected Birth Defects in Hawaii," *American Journal of Epidemiology,* 148, 1998, pp. 1206–1211.

Florack, E. I., G. A. Zielhuis, J. E. Pellegrino, and R. Rolland, "Occupational Physical Activity and the Occurrence of Spontaneous Abortion," *International Journal of Epidemiology,* 22(5), 1993, pp. 878–884.

Frerichs, R. R., "Epidemiologic Monitoring of Possible Health Reactions of Wastewater Reuse," *Science of the Total Environment,* 32, 1984, pp. 353–363.

Frerichs, R. R., K. P. Satin, and E. M. Sloss, *Water Re-use: Its Epidemiologic Impact, Los Angeles County, 1969–71,* Los Angeles: Regents of the University of California, Los Angeles, 1981.

Frerichs, R. R., E. M. Sloss, and K. P. Satin, "Epidemiologic Impact of Water Reuse in Los Angeles County, *Environmental Research,* 29, 1982a, pp. 109–122.

Frerichs, R. R., E. M. Sloss, E. F. Maes, and K. P. Satin, *Water Re-use Part II: Its Epidemiologic Impact, Los Angeles County,* Los Angeles: Regents of the University of California, Los Angeles, 1982b.

Frerichs, R. R., E. M. Sloss, and E. F. Maes, *Water Re-use—Its Epidemiologic Impact Part III, Los Angeles County, 1979–80,* Los Angeles: Regents of the University of California, Los Angeles, 1983.

Froster, U. G., and P. A. Baird, "Maternal Factors, Medications, and Drug Exposure in Congenital Limb Reduction Defects," *Environmental Health Perspectives,* 101, Supplement 3, 1993, pp. 269–274.

Geschwind, S. A., J. A. J. Stolwijk, M. Bracken, et al., "Risk of Congenital Malformations Associated with Proximity of Hazardous Waste," *American Journal of Epidemiology,* 135(11), 1992, pp. 1197–1207.

Goldberg, S. J., M. D. Lebowitz, E. J. Graver, et al., "An Association of Human Congenital Cardiac Malformations and Drinking Water Contaminants," *Journal of the American College of Cardiology,* 16(1), 1990, pp. 155–164.

Hamann, C. L., and B. McEwen, "Potable Water Reuse," in *Municipal Water Reuse: Selected Readings on Water Reuse,* Report No. EPA 430/09-91-022, U.S. Environmental Protection Agency, Washington, D.C., September 1991, pp. 52–58.

Hartikainen, A. L., M. Sorri, H. Anttonen, R. Tuimal, and E. Laara, "Effect of Occupational Noise on the Course and Outcome of Pregnancy," *Scandinavian Journal of Work, Environment and Health,* 20(6), 1994, pp. 444–450.

Hatch, M. S., J. Beyea, J. W. Nieves, et al., "Cancer Near the Three Mile Island Nuclear Plant: Radiation Emissions," *American Journal of Epidemiology,* 132(3), 1990, pp. 397–412.

Healy, D. L., A. O. Trounson, and A. N. Andersen, "Female Infertility: Causes and Treatment," *Lancet,* 343, 1994, pp. 1539–1544.

Hebel, J. R., N. L. Fox, and M. Sexton, "Dose-Response of Birth Weight to Various Measures of Maternal Smoking During Pregnancy," *Journal of Clinical Epidemiology,* 41, 1988, pp. 483–489.

Heinonen, O. P., D. Slone, and S. Shapiro, *Birth Defects and Drugs During Pregnancy,* Littleton, Mass.: Publishing Science Group, 1977.

Hemminki, K., P. Kyyronen, and M. L. Lindbohm, "Spontaneous Abortions and Malformations in the Offspring of Nurses Exposed to Anaesthetic Gases, Cytostatic Drugs, and Other Potential Hazards in Hospitals, Based on Registered Information of Outcome," *Journal of Epidemiology and Community Health,* 39(2), 1985, pp. 141–147.

Hertz-Picciotto, I., S. H. Swan, and R. R. Neutra, "Reporting Bias and Mode of Interview in a Study of Adverse Pregnancy Outcomes and Water Consumption," *Epidemiology,* 3(2), 1992, pp. 104–112.

Hertz-Picciotto, I., S. H. Swan, R. R. Neutra, et al., "Spontaneous Abortions in Relation to Consumption of Tap Water: An Application of Methods from Survival Analysis to a Pregnancy Follow-Up Study," *American Journal of Epidemiology,* 130(1), 1989, pp. 79–93.

Hexter, A. C., J. A. Harris, P. Roeper, L. A. Croen, P. Krueger, and D. Grant, "Evaluation of the Hospital Discharge Diagnoses Index and the Birth Certificate as Sources of Information on Birth Defects," *Public Health Reports,* 105(3), 1990, pp. 296–307.

Hill, A. B., "The Environment and Disease: Association or Causation?" *Proceedings of the Royal Society of Medicine,* 58, 1965, pp. 295–300.

Hyman, I., and G. Dussault, "The Effect of Acculturation on Low Birth Weight in Immigrant Women," *Canadian Journal of Public Health,* (*Revue Canadienne de Sante Publique*), 87(3), 1996, pp. 158–162.

Institute of Medicine (IOM), *Health Consequences of Service During the Persian Gulf War: Recommendations for Research and Information Systems,* Washington, D.C.: National Academy Press, 1996.

John, E. M., D. A. Savitz, and C. M. Shy, "Spontaneous Abortions Among Cosmetologists," *Epidemiology,* 5(2), 1994, pp. 147–155.

Kempe, A., P. H. Wise, N. S. Wampler, F. S. Cole, H. Wallace, C. Dickinson, H. Rinehart, D. C. Lezotte, and B. Beaty, "Risk Status at Discharge and Cause of Death for

Postneonatal Infant Deaths: A Total Population Study," *Pediatrics*, 99(3), 1997, pp. 338–344.

Kessner, David M., James Singer, Carolyn E. Kalk, and Edward R. Schlesinger, *Death: An Analysis by Maternal Risk and Health Care*, Washington, D.C.: Institute of Medicine, National Academy of Sciences, 1973.

Kistin, N., A. Handler, F. Davis, and C. Ferre, "Cocaine and Cigarettes: A Comparison of Risks," *Paediatric and Perinatal Epidemiology*, 10(3), 1996, pp. 269–278.

Kline, J., B. Levin, A. Kinney, Z. Stein, M. Susser, and D. Warburton, "Cigarette Smoking and Spontaneous Abortion of Known Karyotype. Precise Data but Uncertain Inferences," *American Journal of Epidemiology*, 141(5), 1995, pp. 417–427.

Kline, J., Z. Stein, and M. Susser, "Conception to Birth. Epidemiology of Prenatal Development," in *Monographs in Epidemiology and Biostatistics*, Vol. 14, New York: Oxford University Press, 1989.

Klotz, J. B., and L. A. Pyrch, "Neural Tube Defects and Drinking Water Disinfection By-Products," *Epidemiology*, 10(4), 1999, p. 383–390.

Kramer, M. D., C. F. Lynch, P. Isaacson, et al., "The Association of Waterborne Chloroform with Intrauterine Growth Retardation," *Epidemiology*, 3(5), 1992, pp. 407–413.

Kristensen, P., L. M. Irgens, A. K. Daltveit, and A. Andersen, "Perinatal Outcome Among Children of Men Exposed to Lead and Organic Solvents in the Printing Industry," *American Journal of Epidemiology*, 137, 1993, pp. 134–144.

Kurz, H., T. Frischer, W. D. Huber, and M. Gotz, "Adverse Health Effects Caused in Children by Passive Smoking," *Wiener Medizinische Wochenschrift*, 144(22-23), 1994, pp. 531–534.

Kyyronen, P., H. Taskinen, M. L. Lindbohm, K. Hemminki, and O. P. Heinonen, "Spontaneous Abortions and Congenital Malformations Among Women Exposed to Tetrachloroethylene in Dry Cleaning," *Journal of Epidemiology and Community Health*, 43(4), 1989, pp. 346–351.

Lagakos, S. W., B. J. Wessen, and M. Zelen, "An Analysis of Contaminated Well Water and Health Effects in Woburn, MA," *Journal of the American Statistical Association*, 81(395), 1986, pp. 583–596.

Landgren, O., "Environmental Pollution and Delivery Outcome in Southern Sweden: A Study with Central Registries," *Acta Paediatrica*, 85(11), 1996, pp. 1361–1364.

Last, J. M. (ed.), *A Dictionary of Epidemiology*, New York: Oxford University Press, 1983.

Lekea-Karanika, V., and C. Tzoumaka-Bakoula, "Past Obstetric History of the Mother and Its Association with Low Birth Weight of a Subsequent Child: A Population Based Study," *Pediatric and Perinatal Epidemiology*, 8(2), 1994, 173–187.

Li, D. K., J. R. Daling, B. A. Mueller, D. E. Hickok, A. G. Fantel, and N. S. Weiss, "Periconceptional Multivitamin Use in Relation to the Risk of Congenital Urinary Tract Anomalies," *Epidemiology*, 6(3), 1995, pp. 212–218.

Liang, K-Y, and S. L. Zeger, "Longitudinal Analysis for Generalized Linear Models," *Biometrika*, 73, 1986, pp. 13–22.

Lieberman, E., I. Gremy, J. M. Lang, and A. P. Cohen, "Low Birth Weight at Term and the Timing of Fetal Exposure to Maternal Smoking," *American Journal of Public Health*, 84(7), 1994, pp. 1127–1131.

Lin, S., E. G. Marshall, and G. K. Davidson, "Potential Parental Exposure to Pesticides and Limb Reduction Defects," *Scandinavian Journal of Work, Environment and Health*, 20(3), 1994, pp. 166–179.

Lopez-Camelo, J. S., and I. M. Orioli, "Heterogeneous Rates for Birth Defects in Latin America: Hints on Causality," *Genetic Epidemiology*, 13(5), 1996, pp. 469–481.

Lowe, C. R., C. J. Roberts, and S. Lloyd, "Malformations of Central Nervous System and Softness of Local Water Supplies," *British Medical Journal*, (2), 1971, pp. 357–361.

Lynberg, M. C., M. J. Khoury, X. Lu, and T. Cocian, "Maternal Flu, Fever, and the Risk of Neural Tube Defects: A Population-Based Case-Control Study," *American Journal of Epidemiology*, 140(3), 1994, pp. 244–255.

Marshall, E. G., L. Gensburg, E. Deres, et al., "Maternal Residential Exposure to Hazardous Wastes and Risk of Central Nervous System and Musculoskeletal Birth Defects," *Archives of Environmental Health*, 52(6), 1997. pp. 416–425.

Mastroiacovo, P., C. Corchia, L. D. Botto, R. Lanni, G. Zampino, and D. Fusco, "Epidemiology and Genetics of Microtia-Anotia: A Registry Based Study on Over One Million Births," *Journal of Medical Genetics*, 32(6), 1995, pp. 453–457.

Matte, T. D., J. Mulinare, and J. D. Erickson, "Case Control Study of Congenital Defects and Parental Employment in Health Care," *American Journal of Industrial Medicine*, 24(1), 1993, pp. 11–23.

McMichael, A. J., G. V. Vimpani, E. F. Robertson, P. A. Baghurst, and P. D. Clark, "The Port Pirie Cohort Study: Maternal Blood Lead and Pregnancy Outcome," *Journal of Epidemiology and Community Health*, 40(1), 1986, pp. 18–25.

Montebello Forebay Groundwater Recharge Engineering Report, "Sanitation Districts of Los Angeles County, Los Angeles County Department of Public Works, and the Water Replenishment District of Southern California," November 1997.

Mor, J. M., G. R. Alexander, M. D. Kogan, E. C. Kieffer, and H. M. Ichiho, "Similarities and Disparities in Maternal Risk and Birth Outcomes of White and Japanese-American Mothers," *Paediatric and Perinatal Epidemiology*, 9(1), 1995, pp. 59–73.

Morgan, H. V., memorandum to Elizabeth Sloss, "Water Quality of Domestic Supplies Served Within the Pomona Valley by the City of Pomona," March 3, 1994a.

Morgan, H. V., memorandum to Elizabeth Sloss, "Water Quality of Domestic Supplies Served Within the San Fernando Valley by the City of Los Angeles," March 3, 1994b.

Morgan, H. V., memorandum to Elizabeth Sloss, "Water Quality of Domestic Supplies Served Within the City of San Fernando," March 3, 1994c.

Morgenstern, H., "Uses of Ecologic Analysis in Epidemiologic Research," *American Journal of Public Health*, 72(12), 1982, pp. 1336–1344.

Morton, M. S., P. C. Elwood, and M. Abernathy, "Trace Elements in Water and Congenital Malformations of the Central Nervous System in South Wales," *British Journal of Preventive and Social Medicine*, 30, 1976, pp. 36–39.

National Research Council (NRC), *Issues in Potable Reuse: The Viability of Augmenting Drinking Water Supplies with Reclaimed Water*, Washington, D.C.: National Academy Press, 1998.

Nellor, M. H., R. B. Baird, and J. R. Smyth, *Summary of Health Effects Study: Final Report*, County Sanitation Districts of Los Angeles County, Whittier, California, March 1984.

Neugebauer, R., J. Kline, Z. Stein, P. Shrout, D. Warburton, and M. Susser, "Association of Stressful Life Events with Chromosomally Normal Spontaneous Abortion," *American Journal of Epidemiology*, 143(6), 1996, pp. 588–596.

Neutra, R. R., S. H. Swan, I. Hertz-Picciotto, G. C. Windham, M. Wrensch, G. M. Shaw, L. Fenster, and M. Deane, "Potential Sources of Bias and Confounding in Environmental Epidemiologic Studies of Pregnancy Outcomes," *Epidemiology*, 1992, pp. 134–142.

Norska-Borowka, I., "Pediatric Problems in Upper Silesia—Region of Ecological Disaster," *Toxicology Letters*, 72(1-3), 1994, pp. 219–225.

Nurminen, T., "Female Noise Exposure, Shift Work, and Reproduction," *Journal of Occupational and Environmental Medicine*, 37(8), 1995, pp. 945–950.

Olshan, A. F., and E. M. Faustmann, "Male-Mediated Developmental Toxicity," *Annual Review Public Health*, 14, 1993, pp. 159–181.

Olshan, A. F., T. Kay, and P. A. Baird, "Birth Defects Among Offspring of Firemen," *American Journal of Epidemiology*, 131, 1990, pp. 312–320.

Olshan, A. F., K. Teschke, and P. A. Baird, "Paternal Occupation and Congenital Anomalies in Offspring," *American Journal of Industrial Medicine*, 20, 1991, pp. 447–475.

Orr, S. T., S. A. James, C. A. Miller, B. Barakat, N. Daikoku, M. Pupkin, K. Engstrom, and G. Huggins, "Psychosocial Stressors and Low Birth Weight in an Urban Population," *American Journal of Preventive Medicine*, 12(6), 1996, pp. 459–466.

Parazzini, F., L. Luchini, C. La Vecchia, and P. G. Crosignani, "Video Display Terminal Use During Pregnancy and Reproductive Outcome—A Meta-Analysis," *Journal of Epidemiology and Community Health,* 47(4), 1993, pp. 265–268.

Penrose, L. S., "Genetics of Anencephaly," *Journal of Mental Deficiency Research,* 1(4), 1957.

Pickering, R. M., "Relative Risks of Low Birth Weight in Scotland 1980–2," *Journal of Epidemiology and Community Health,* 41(2), 1987, pp. 133–139.

Polissar, L., "The Effect of Migration on Comparison of Disease Rates in Geographic Studies in the United States," *American Journal of Epidemiology,* 111, 1980, pp. 175–182.

Pradat, P., "Recurrence Risk for Major Congenital Heart Defects in Sweden: A Registry Study," *Genetic Epidemiology,* 11(2), 1994, pp. 131–140.

Prentice, R. L., and L. P. Zhao, "Estimating Equations for Parameters in Means and Covariances of Multivariate Discrete and Continuous Responses," *Biometrics,* 47, 1991, pp. 825–839.

Reif, J. S., M. C. Hatch, M. Bracken, L. B. Holmes, B. A. Schwetz, and P. C. Singer, "Reproductive and Developmental Effects of Disinfection By-Products in Drinking Water," *Environmental Health Perspectives,* 104(10), 1996, pp. 1056–1061.

Riedmiller, K., and S. Ficenec, "Vital Statistics of California 1992," Department of Health Services, State of California, December 1994.

Risch, H. A., N. S. Weiss, E. A. Clarke, and A. B. Miller, "Risk Factors for Spontaneous Abortion and Its Recurrence," *American Journal of Epidemiology,* 128(2), 1988, pp. 420–430.

Robeck, G. G., K. P. Cantor, R. F. Christman, et al., *Report of the Scientific Advisory Panel on Groundwater Recharge with Reclaimed Wastewater,* prepared for State of California, State Water Resources Control Board, Department of Water Resources, Department of Health Services, November 1987.

Rodriguez, C., E. Regidor, and J. L. Gutierrez-Fisac, "Low Birth Weight in Spain Associated with Sociodemographic Factors," *Journal of Epidemiology and Community Health,* 49(1), 1995, pp. 38–42.

Rothman, K. J., *Modern Epidemiology,* Boston: Little, Brown and Company, 1986.

Rowland, A. S., D. D. Baird, D. L. Shore, B. Darden, and A. J. Wilcox, "Ethylene Oxide Exposure May Increase the Risk of Spontaneous Abortion, Preterm Birth, and Postterm Birth," *Epidemiology,* 7(4), pp. 363–368.

Rowland, A. S., D. D. Baird, D. L. Shore, C. R. Weinberg, D. A. Savitz, and A. J. Wilcox, "Nitrous Oxide and Spontaneous Abortion in Female Dental Assistants," *American Journal of Epidemiology,* 141(6), 1995, pp. 531–538.

Savitz, D. A., K. W. Andrews, and L. M. Pastore, "Drinking Water and Pregnancy Outcome in Central North Carolina: Source, Amount, and Trihalomethane Levels," *Environmental Health Perspectives*, 103(6), 1995, pp. 592–596.

Savitz, D., and C. L. Moe, "Water: Chlorinated Hydrocarbons and Infectious Agents," in N. K. Steenland and D. A. Savitz, eds., *Topics in Environmental Epidemiology*, New York: Oxford University Press, 1997, pp. 89–118.

Schieve, L. A., A. Handler, R. Hershow, V. Persky, and F. Davis, "Urinary Tract Infection During Pregnancy: Its Association with Maternal Morbidity and Perinatal Outcome," *American Journal of Public Health*, 84(3), 1994, pp. 405–410.

Schnitzer, P. G., A. F. Olshan, and J. D. Erickson, "Paternal Occupation and Risk of Birth Defects in Offspring," *Epidemiology*, 6(6), 1995, pp. 577–583.

Schrader, S. M., and J. S. Kesner, "Male Reproductive Toxicology," in M. Paul, ed., *Occupational and Environmental Hazards: A Guide for Clinicians*, Baltimore, Md.: Williams and Wilkins, 1993.

Schwartz, D. A., L. A. Newsum, and R. M. Heifetz, "Parental Occupation and Birth Outcome in an Agricultural Community," *Scandinavian Journal of Work, Environment and Health*, 12(1), pp. 51–54.

Scialli, A. R., *A Clinical Guide to Reproductive and Developmental Toxicology*, Boca Raton, Fla.: CRC Press, 1992.

Scragg, R. K. R., M. M. Dorsch, A. J. McMichael, et al., "Birth Defects and Household Water Supply: Epidemiologic Studies in the Mount Gambier Region of South Australia," *The Medical Journal of Australia*, 25, 1982, pp. 577–579.

Shah, B. V., B. G. Barnwell, and G. S. Bieler, *SUDAAN User's Manual, Release 7.5*, Research Triangle Park, N.C.: Research Triangle Institute, 1997.

Sharma, R., C. Synkewecz, T. Raggio, and D. R. Mattison, "Intermediate Variables as Determinants of Adverse Pregnancy Outcome in High-Risk Inner-City Populations," *Journal of the National Medical Association*, 86(11), 1994, pp. 857–860.

Shaw, G. M., and L. H. Malcoe, "Residential Mobility During Pregnancy for Mothers of Infants With or Without Congenital Cardiac Anomalies," *Archives of Environmental Health*, 46, 1991, pp. 310–312.

Shaw, G. M., S. H. Swan, J. A. Harris, et al., "Maternal Water Consumption During Pregnancy and Congenital Cardiac Anomalies," *Epidemiology*, 1(3), 1990, pp. 206–210.

Shepard, T. H., *Catalog of Teratogenic Agents*, Seventh Edition, Baltimore, Md.: The Johns Hopkins University Press, 1992.

Shiota, K., "Maternal Fertility, Reproductive Loss, and Defective Human Embryos," *Journal of Epidemiology and Community Health*, 43(3), 1989, pp. 261–267.

Singh, G. K., and S. M. Yu, "Adverse Pregnancy Outcomes: Differences Between US- and Foreign-Born Women in Major US Racial and Ethnic Groups," *American Journal of Public Health,* 86(6), 1996, pp. 837–843.

Singh, G. K., and S. M. Yu, "Birth Weight Differentials Among Asian Americans," *American Journal of Public Health,* 84(9), 1994, pp. 1444–1449.

Skakkebaek, N. E., A. Giwercman, and D. de Kretser, "Pathogenesis and Management of Male Infertility," *Lancet,* 343, 1994, pp. 1473–1479.

Sloss, E. M., S. A. Geschwind, D. F. McCaffrey, and B. R. Ritz, *Groundwater Recharge with Reclaimed Water: An Epidemiologic Assessment in Los Angeles County, 1987–1991,* Santa Monica, Calif.: RAND, MR-679-WRDSC, 1996.

Snedecor, G. W., and W. G. Cochran, *Statistical Methods,* Ames, Iowa: The Iowa State University Press, 1989.

Sosniak, W. A., W. E. Kaye, and T. M. Gomez, "Data Linkage to Explore the Risk of Low Birth Weight Associated with Maternal Proximity to Hazardous Waste Sites from the National Priorities List," *Archives of Environmental Health,* 49(4), 1994, pp. 251–255.

"Spontaneous Abortion in a Hospital Population: Are Tobacco and Coffee Intake Risk Factors?" *European Journal of Epidemiology,* 10(6), 1994, pp. 665–668.

Sram, R. J., I. Benes, B. Binkova, J. Dejmek, D. Horstman, F. Kotesovec, D. Otto, S. D. Perreault, J. Rubes, S. G. Selevan, et al., "Teplice Program—The impact of Air Pollution on Human Health," *Environmental Health Perspectives,* 104, Supplement 4, 1996, pp. 699–714.

Stierman, L., *Birth Defects in California, 1983–1990,* Emeryville, Calif.: California Birth Defects Monitoring Program, 1994.

St. Leger, A. S., P. C. Elwood, and M. S. Morton, "Neural Tube Malformations and Trace Elements in Water," *Journal of Epidemiology and Community Health,* 34, 1980, pp. 186–187.

Stoll, C., Y. Alembik, B. Dott, and M. P. Roth, "An Epidemiologic Study of Environmental and Genetic Factors in Congenital Hydrocephalus," *European Journal of Epidemiology,* 8(6), 1992, pp. 797–803.

Stoltenberg, C., P. Magnus, R. T. Lie, A. K. Daltveit, and L. M. Irgens, "Birth Defects and Parental Consanguinity in Norway," *American Journal of Epidemiology,* 145(5), 1997, pp. 439–448.

Sullivan, F. M., "Impact of the Environment on Reproduction from Conception to Parturition," *Environmental Health Perspectives,* 101, Supplement 2, 1993, pp. 13–18.

Susser, M., W. A. Hauser, J. L. Kiely, N. Paneth, and Z. Stein, "Quantitative Estimates of Prenatal and Perinatal Risk Factors for Perinatal Mortality, Cerebral Palsy, Mental Retardation, and Epilepsy," in J. M. Freeman, ed., *Prenatal and Perinatal*

Factors Associated with Brain Disorders, Bethesda, Md.: NIH Publication No. 85-1149, 1985, pp. 359–439.

Swan, S. H., R. R. Neutra, M. Wrensch, I. Hertz-Picciotto, G. C. Windham, L. Fenster, D. M. Epstein, and M. Deane, "Is Drinking Water Related to Spontaneous Abortion? Reviewing the Evidence from the California Department of Health Services Studies," *Epidemiology,* 3(2), 1992, pp. 83–93.

Swan, S. H., G. Shaw, J. A. Harris, et al., "Congenital Cardiac Anomalies in Relation to Water Contamination, Santa Clara County, California, 1981–1983," *American Journal of Epidemiology,* 129, 1989, pp. 885–893.

Swan, S. H., K. Waller, B. Hopkins, G. Windham, L. Fenster, C. Schaefer, and R. R. Neutra, "A Prospective Study of Spontaneous Abortion: Relation to Amount and Source of Drinking Water Consumed in Early Pregnancy," *Epidemiology,* 9, 1998, 126–133.

Thomas, D. C., J. Siemiatycki, R. Dewar, et al., "The Problem of Multiple Inference in Studies Designed to Generate Hypotheses," *American Journal of Epidemiology,* 122, 1985, pp. 1080–1095.

Tikkanen, J., and O. P. Heinonen, "Risk Factors for Atrial Septal Defect," *European Journal of Epidemiology,* 8(4), 1992a, pp. 509–515.

Tikkanen, J., and O. P. Heinonen, "Risk Factors for Conal Malformations of the Heart," *European Journal of Epidemiology,* 8(1), 1992b, pp. 48–57.

Tikkanen, J., and O. P. Heinonen, "Risk Factors for Hypoplastic Left Heart Syndrome," *Teratology,* 50(2), 1994, pp. 112–117.

Waller, K., S. H. Swan, G. DeLorenze, and B. Hopkins, "Trihalomethanes in Drinking Water and Spontaneous Abortion," *Epidemiology,* 9, 1998, pp. 134–140.

Weinberg, C. R., I. Hertz-Picciotto, D. D. Baird, and A. J. Wilcox, "Efficiency and Bias in Studies of Early Pregnancy Loss," *Epidemiology,* 3, 1992, pp. 17–22.

Weinberg, C. R., R. Skjaerven, and A. J. Wilcox, "Statistical Evidence for Shared Transient Causes of Anatomically Distinct Birth Defects," *Statistics in Medicine,* 15, 1996, pp. 2029–2036.

Weisberg, S., *Applied Linear Regression,* 2nd ed., New York: John Wiley & Sons, 1985.

Werler, M. M., A. A. Mitchell, and S. Shapiro, "Demographic, Reproductive, Medical, and Environmental Factors in Relation to Gastroschisis," *Teratology,* 45(4), 1992, pp. 353–360.

Werler, M. M., S. Shapiro, and A. A. Mitchell, "Periconceptional Folic Acid Exposure and Risk of Occurrent Neural Tube Defects," *Journal of the American Medical Association,* 269(10), 1993, pp. 1257–1261.

Windham, G. C., S. H. Swan, L. Fenster, and R. R. Neutra, "Tap or Bottled Water Consumption and Spontaneous Abortion: A 1986 Case-Control Study in California," *Epidemiology*, 3(2), 1992, pp. 113–119.

World Health Organization, *International Classification of Diseases: Manual of the International Statistical Classification of Diseases, Injuries and Causes of Death*, Ninth Revision, Geneva, Switzerland: World Health Organization, 1977.

Wrensch, M., S. H. Swan, J. Lipscomb, et al., "Pregnancy Outcomes in Women Potentially Exposed to Solvent-Contaminated Drinking Water in San Jose, California," *American Journal of Epidemiology*, 131, 1990, pp. 283–300.

Wrensch, M., S. H. Swan, J. Lipscomb, et al., "Spontaneous Abortions and Birth Defects Related to Tap and Bottled Water Use, San Jose, California, 1980–1985," *Epidemiology*, 3(2), 1992, pp. 98–103.

Xu, X., M. Ding, B. Li, and D. C. Christiani, "Association of Rotating Shiftwork with Preterm Births and Low Birth Weight Among Never Smoking Women Textile Workers in China," *Occupational and Environmental Medicine*, 51(7), 1994, pp. 470–474.

Yen, I. H., M. J. Khoury, J. D. Erickson, et al., "The Changing Epidemiology of Neural Tube Defects, United States, 1968–1989," *American Journal of Diseases of Children*, 146, 1992, pp. 857–861.

Zhang, H., and M. B. Bracken, "Tree-Based, Two-Stage Risk Factor Analysis for Spontaneous Abortion," *American Journal of Epidemiology*, 144(10), 1996, pp. 989–996.

Zhang, J., and J. M. Ratcliffe, "Paternal Smoking and Birth Weight in Shanghai," *American Journal of Public Health*, 83(2), 1993, pp. 207–210.

Zierler, S., A. Cohen, and K. J. Rothman, "Chemical Quality of Maternal Drinking Water and Congenital Heart Disease," *International Journal of Epidemiology*, 17(3), 1988, pp. 589–594.